The editors of **Prevention**®

DON'T GET SICK.

A PANIC-FREE POCKET GUIDE TO LIVING IN A GERM-FILLED WORLD!

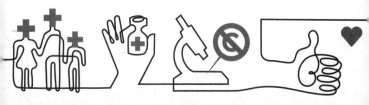

© 2010 by Rodale Inc.

Illustrations © 2010 by Felix Sockwell

Book design by Susan Eugster

Contributing writers: Elizabeth Shimer Bowers, Sandra Salera-Lloyd, Eric Metcalf, Joely Johnson Mork, Wyatt Myers, Linda Rao, Maureen Sangiorgio, and Marie Suszynski

Library of Congress Cataloging-in-Publication Data is on file with publisher.

ISBN 13: 978-1-60529-423-0

Distributed to the trade by Macmillan

2 4 6 8 10 9 7 5 3 1   paperback

LIVE YOUR WHOLE LIFE™

We inspire and enable people to improve their lives and the world around them

For more of our products visit **rodalestore.com** or call 800-848-4735

To your best health

Contents

Introduction vi

Introduction

Every once in a while, Mother Nature likes to throw a new disease outbreak our way, maybe just to keep us on our toes. In 2004 SARS (short for severe acute respiratory syndrome) took the world stage; that same year, and again 2 years later, avian flu made international headlines. Now we're facing another formidable infectious foe in the form of H1N1, the so-called swine flu.

What makes these bugs so scary is that we don't know very much about them—unlike, say, seasonal flu, whose annual appearance is comparable to crabby Aunt Martha showing up for Thanksgiving dinner. You can't do anything to stop either one from coming, so you prepare as best as you can while telling yourself that it will be over soon. At least you can get a vaccine against seasonal flu; with Aunt Martha, you're on your own.

Whether it's seasonal flu or something more serious that's lurking, this idea of getting ready—but not going overboard—makes good sense. As you'll discover in the pages ahead, you can do a lot to safeguard yourself against the viruses, bacteria, and other disease-causing microbes that want nothing more than to make themselves at home inside your body. We're talking simple things, like eating lunch away from your desk (it's germier than a toilet seat!), stowing your purse or briefcase off the floor, and microwaving your kitchen sponge.

It's true that you may not be able to avoid germs completely. But you can reduce your exposure and strengthen your immunity—one small change at a time.

—*The editors of Prevention*

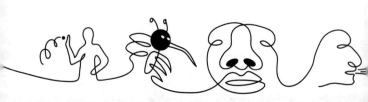

MEET YOUR IMMUNE SYSTEM

A GOOD OFFENSE IS THE BEST DEFENSE

Considering that some 500 million rhinoviruses—the culprit behind the common cold—can fit on the head of a pin, it's an understatement to say that we humans are outnumbered by the disease-causing microorganisms in our environment.

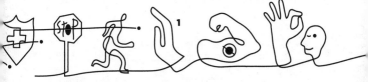

That we don't get sick more often is pretty amazing. We have our immune systems to thank.

You might think of your immune system as your body's own personal Secret Service detail. While you're going about your business, it's keeping an eye out for viruses, bacteria, and other disease-causing microbes. When it spies a potential troublemaker, it radios for backup, in the form of immune-cell specialists that surround and take down the suspect organisms. And it's on alert 24–7.

Most germs aren't wily enough to outsmart this sophisticated system. But every once in a while, one of them evades detection. A virus, for example, can masquerade as an acceptable substance or take cover inside or between red blood cells. If it's *novel*, meaning that your immune system hasn't encountered it

RealityCheck ✔+

If you go outside with wet hair, you'll get sick.

The wet hair alone won't make you sick, says Erika Schwartz, MD, chief medical officer of www.healthandprevention.com. But the combination of cold air temperature and wet hair can lower your immunity and make you more vulnerable to viruses and bacteria. On the other hand, warming up your extremities—especially your head—helps support your immune system.

So while medical science hasn't directly linked any health risks to going outside with wet hair, there's really no good reason to do it. As Dr. Schwartz says, "Why take the risk if the solution is as simple as taking a few minutes to dry your hair?"

before, it's more likely to slip past unnoticed.

Sometimes the immune system itself isn't operating up to snuff. Poor eating and lifestyle habits, chronic disease, and even age can take a toll. You might not be able to change your age (if only!), but you can do a lot to reinforce and strengthen your immune function, as you'll see in the chapters ahead. A robust immune system is still your best defense against infection. Then germs will have to find someplace else to do their dirty work.

White (Blood Cell) in Shining Armor

At any moment, your body is under assault from countless microorganisms that want to cause harm. Often they gain entry through tiny cuts and abrasions in your skin or through natural portals like your nasal passageways. Once inside, each kind of organism has its own modus operandi. But not to worry: Your immune system is ready to respond.

What may be most impressive about your immune system is its ability to distinguish friend (that is, your own cells) from foe (viruses and bacteria, for example). Your cells carry markers that act as biochemical ID cards, allowing your immune system to recognize them as official members of the club known as your body. Those substances without markers are called antigens. Their lack of proper ID draws the attention of your immune system, which quickly dispatches leukocytes to investigate the intruders.

Leukocytes are white blood cells that take several different forms, each with a particular disease-fighting skill. Some are adept at recogniz-

(continued on page 6)

Know the Lingo

As you read about infectious illness in this book and elsewhere, you'll come across terminology that—let's face it—doesn't exactly put your mind at ease. H1N1? Sounds like a top-secret government project. Outbreak? Could be the title of a science-fiction movie.

Simply getting a handle on what these terms mean can offset the fear factor and give proper perspective to all the hyperbolic headlines. Here's a glossary to help.

Avian flu
An influenza-A virus that occurs naturally among wild birds. Some strains don't cause major problems, while others—such as H5N1, which can spread from birds to humans—can be quite serious. Generally, the risk to humans is low. Symptoms are similar to seasonal flu, though complications such as pneumonia and acute respiratory disease have been reported.

Epidemic
The spread of a disease within a specific region or country.

Influenza virus
A virus that causes influenza. There are three types: A, which is prevalent in humans and animals such as birds, pigs, and whales; B, which occurs only in humans; and C, found in humans, pigs, and dogs. Type C usually doesn't cause outbreaks.

MRSA (pronounced "MER-sa")
Short for methicillin-resistant *Staphylococcus aureus,* a bacterium that causes staph infection. As its name suggests, it resists treatment with several common antibiotics. MRSA commonly occurs in hospital settings, though it can pass from one person to another through skin-to-skin contact.

Outbreak
The spread of a disease over a short period of time in a specific region.

Pandemic

The spread of a viral disease across a large geographic area that meets these three criteria:

✚ The virus is new, and the human body hasn't developed a natural immunity to it.

✚ The virus causes serious illness.

✚ The virus spreads easily among populations.

Seasonal flu

A contagious respiratory illness caused by various types of influenza virus; also called the common flu, or just "the flu." People can contract seasonal flu up to 4 days before symptoms appear. Healthy adults are infectious from the day before symptoms appear until 5 to 7 days after. Symptoms include headaches, fever, dry cough, and body aches. While seasonal flu can be serious, most people recover in 1 to 2 weeks.

Swine flu (H1N1)

An influenza-A virus first seen in the United States in April 2009 and classified as a pandemic 2 months later. Initial testing suggested that H1N1 was similar to a virus spread among pigs (hence the name swine flu). Subsequent lab results showed that it was a mix of genes from swine, bird, and human viruses. Symptoms are similar to the common flu, although there have been reports of nausea, vomiting, and diarrhea, which are rarely seen with seasonal flu.

Vaccine

A product of weakened or killed viruses or bacteria that stimulates the immune system to produce antibodies. A vaccine can be administered as a shot (inoculation) or as nasal spray.

Virus

A tiny parasite consisting of either RNA or DNA and surrounded by a protein coat. Viruses invade healthy cells to survive and reproduce.

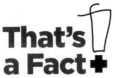

That's a Fact

Airplanes are dirtier than public toilets.

Planes don't get cleaned very often, and the scientific data on the number of viruses and bacteria per square inch is horrifying, says Erika Schwartz, MD, chief medical officer of www.healthandprevention.com. When you travel by air, take steps to keep germs from hitching a ride on the friendly skies. Wash your hands often, and wipe down your seat and tray with disinfectant wipes.

ing and destroying foreign substances, while others form antibodies to them. If and when an antigen attempts a return appearance, antibodies will promptly escort them from your body.

Your immune system also comes equipped with its very own circulatory system, called the lymphatic system. It's an elaborate highway of vessels that branch out into all of the tissues of your body, just like blood vessels. The key difference is that lymphatic vessels carry lymph fluid—the leukocytes' primary means of transport—instead of blood.

All along the lymphatic route are rest stops of lymph glands and lymph nodes that house leukocytes and produce lymph fluid. So no matter where or how a foreign substance enters your body, leukocytes can be on the scene in a flash, before the microbe can do harm.

A Virus-Eye View

To help illustrate just how your immune system works, let's tag along with an influenza virus as it attempts to run the gauntlet of immune defenses, as it must do before it can sideline you with the flu.

First, of course, it needs to get inside your body. The most likely route is through your nose and throat, as a sneeze or cough from someone who's infected sends viral particles parachuting through the air—and you inhale them. Once it gains entry, it scouts around for a healthy cell whose internal machinery it can essentially hijack for its own growth and reproduction.

But your body is already fighting back. Let's say the virus came in through your nose. In doing so, it tripped a respiratory alarm of sorts, causing the nasal passageways to ramp up their production of mucus to trap the virus. Then cilia—the fine hairs that line your respiratory tract—move the mucus away from your lungs. This triggers a sneezing or coughing reflex, as your body attempts to get rid of the virus for good.

Does it work?

Airborne

Worth a try

Developed by a second-grade schoolteacher, Airborne is a tablet combination of 17 herbs, minerals, and vitamins that claims to support the immune system. Ingredients include vitamins A, C, and E; the minerals zinc, selenium, manganese, and magnesium; amino acids; and a special proprietary herbal blend.

"Airborne alone probably isn't going to keep you from getting sick," says Erika Schwartz, MD, chief medical officer of www.healthand prevention.com. "I don't use it personally, but it isn't dangerous. When used with other immune-boosting measures, it can't hurt."

That's a Fact

If the virus manages to survive this initial blitz, it must then navigate your respiratory passages to reach the target cell. Getting through any passageway in your body is no easy task. The respiratory, digestive, and urogenital tracts are coated with mucus to protect the layers of cells underneath. These mucosal surfaces also secrete a special kind of antibody called IgA (short for immunoglobulin A). The mission of IgA is to keep the virus from attaching to the cell surface.

Remember those leukocytes we talked about earlier? This is where they come into play. If the virus manages to elude IgA, the leukocytes step up to finish off the bug once and for all.

There are several different categories of leukocytes, each with a very specific role. Phagocytes, for example, are large white blood cells with a voracious appetite. They like to ingest foreign substances of all kinds, including viruses.

T cells are a bit more particular. These small but potent white blood cells are equipped with keylike receptors that match specific antigens. If the virus fits its receptor exactly, the T cell sounds the alarm. Then other immune cells rush in to ambush the suspect organism.

Some T cells, called helper T cells, help direct and regulate the immune response. They work closely with B cells, which secrete a cocktail of antibodies made precisely for a particular virus. Other T cells, the killer T cells, can wipe out any infected cells.

Both T and B cells have an extraordinary memory. When they meet a substance that they've never encountered before, they remember its genetic composition so they can identify and attack it faster the next time. This is what's known as acquired immunity. Vaccinations work on the same principle: Introducing a small amount of a disease-causing microorganism (or its derivative) to the body stimulates production of antibodies that can help fend off the germ should it try to gain a foothold again.

That's a Fact

Handbags, suitcases, and briefcases can be as dirty as the soles of your shoes. Think about it: You routinely set these items on restroom floors, store counters, maybe even on sidewalks and streets. So keep them away from anything that eventually could come near your nose or mouth, advises Sue DeCotiis, MD, a board-certified internal medicine specialist in private practice in New York City. "When guests enter my home, I immediately invite them to leave their handbags or briefcases on a shelf in the hall," she says.

As much as we know about the immune system, we still have much more to learn. Why, for instance, does it sometimes go rogue and tag normally harmless substances like pollen as antigens? How can we harness and direct its remarkable protective powers to fight diseases besides the infectious kind?

They're huge questions, the answers to which could fill a book (or two!). For our purposes, what matters most is this: Your immune system is your best protection against colds, flu, and other bugs, and you can keep it in disease-fighting form with good, basic self-care. We'll show you how!

The Pros Know

James Beckerman, MD

Heart expert for WebMD, a cardiologist at the Providence Heart and Vascular Institute, and author of The Single Pound Solution

As a physician and father of two toddlers in day care, Dr. Beckerman gets a daily dose of viruses and bacteria. Here's what he does to fend them off.

Health-care providers are in a unique situation because they need to stay healthy for their patients as well as for themselves. To keep myself as healthy as possible, I get plenty of sleep (when not on call, of course!), exercise regularly, and go easy on caffeine.

Having two toddlers makes all of the above more challenging—not to mention the germs they bring home from day care. We try to make sure the kids keep their hands clean and stay away from diaper pails and garbage cans that can put them at risk. When they are sick, though, it's hard to avoid close contact, so we do what we can to boost our immune systems.

At work, I always wash my hands and use hand sanitizer outside patient rooms. I realize that stethoscopes can carry as many germs as elevator buttons, so I try to clean mine frequently. I also make sure my sicker patients are gowned and gloved, even for simple contact. And I cannot overemphasize the importance of flu shots—for health-care providers, children, and everyone else.

2

HOW GERM-SAVVY ARE YOU?

MAKE THE MOST OF YOUR HYGIENE M.O.

Not to freak you out or anything, but you're crawling with bacteria.

When researchers at the National Institutes of Health studied samples from 20 different skin sites, they identified as many as 205 unique genera of bacteria. (Genera are classifications of living

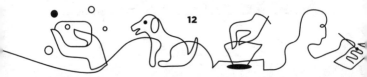

organisms.) Some 44 species make themselves at home on your forearm. Another 19 species hang out behind your ears. (So that's why mom made you wash back there!)

Your reaction to this bit of science reveals a lot about how you might cope when germs run amok, whether you're facing yet another cold and flu season or an unexpected outbreak of an unfamiliar illness. As much as you might like to, you just can't avoid germs completely. They vastly outnumber us, for one thing. For another, they're incredibly resilient, having been around for the past 250 million years or so—way longer than we humans.

In fairness to our microscopic cohabitants, they aren't all bad. Actually, our survival as a species to a large degree depends on their presence. Take *Lactobacillus acidophilus*, for instance. These bacteria reside in your gut, where they aid your digestion and support your immune function. Cyanobacteria, found in the ocean, generate the oxygen you breathe. The fungus *Arbuscular mycorrhiza* helps plants process nutrients from the soil—nutrients that

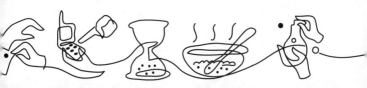

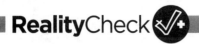

RealityCheck

Chicken soup is nature's best cold and flu remedy.

Although chicken soup probably doesn't kill viruses, it's such a common cold and flu remedy around the world that there must be something to its therapeutic power.

"A number of years ago, the Israelis invented an interesting soup-drinking cup with a spout that bent around it, practically causing the soup to go up your nose when you drink it," notes Margaret Lewin, MD, clinical assistant professor of medicine at Cornell University and chief medical director of Cinergy Health. "I think that the warmth and steam from the soup help. And it's a good source of protein. Plus, chicken soup is liquid, and you really need fluids to stay hydrated when you're sick."

eventually find their way to you, through food.

Even viruses have some redeeming qualities. For example, they're instrumental in the search for new medical treatments. Scientists are using viruses to kill harmful bacteria, explore gene therapies, and clone DNA.

So even if you could somehow fashion a microbe-free existence for yourself, you wouldn't necessarily want to. On the other hand, you don't want your habits to aid and abet the viruses, bacteria, and other pathogens that are just itching to infect you (and everyone around you).

We've put together this short self-test to help you find out where you fall on the germophobe-germophile scale. Simply read the question, then choose the answer that seems to best suit you. Our completely unofficial, though not entirely unscientific, assessment of your answers follows next.

Your Hygiene M.O.

1 You've just used a public restroom. Before you leave, you:

a. Scrub your hands for at least 1 minute with antibacterial soap that you carry with you at all times, dry your hands with paper towels, use another towel to open the restroom door, and then rub sanitizer on your hands for good measure.

b. Wash your hands with soap and water and dry your hands with paper towels.

c. Check yourself in the mirror.

✚ Most people would say that the germiest place they visit with some regularity is a public restroom. Just imagine the microbes crawling on all of those surfaces—door handles, toilet seats, counters, faucet handles, and soap dispensers. In a telephone survey of 1,001 people, 92 percent said that they washed their hands after using a public bathroom. However, in an observational study conducted in four major cities, only 77 percent were seen washing their hands.

And men were far less meticulous than women: Just 66 percent of men lathered up, compared to 88 percent of women. At one sporting event at Turner Field in Atlanta, only 57 percent of men washed their hands. Atlanta truly is home of the Brave!

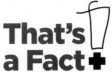

That's a Fact ✚

If your hand sanitizer dries in less than 20 seconds, you're not using enough. For a hand sanitizer to be effective, you need to do the same thing that you would if you were washing your hands at the sink, says Margaret Lewin, MD, clinical assistant professor of medicine at Cornell University and chief medical director of Cinergy Health. "Really wash well between your fingers, under your nails, and on the backs of your hands and the lower part of your wrists," she advises.

2 Your friend's Saint Bernard puppy gives you a sloppy kiss on the hand. You:

a. Shoo the dog away, break out the sanitizer, and vigorously rub your hands together, all while discreetly suppressing the urge to vomit.

b. Give the dog a playful pat on the head or scratch under the chin and wash your hands with soap and water shortly after.

c. Give him a sloppy smooch right back, shake his paw, and scratch his belly before diving into the chips and dip.

✚ "He who lies down with dogs shall rise up with fleas," as the saying goes—but that doesn't mean he (or she) is any more likely to get sick. According to researchers at Kansas State College of Veterinary Medicine, sharing a bed and sharing food with your pet doesn't ramp up your risk of illness. Not washing up after a lick from Fido or Fluffy is a bit dicier. Dog and cat saliva harbor more than 100 different germs that they can pass along to you. So give your pets all the attention and affection they deserve—then wash your hands before you do one other thing! The same rule applies when cleaning your cat's litter box or your dog's poop.

3 Your boss has a terrible cold—watery eyes, runny nose, a hacking cough, and chapped lips. She stops by your desk to go over a report and sneezes in your direction. You:

a. Quit on the spot.

b. Offer her a tissue and then continue your chat.

c. Loan her your ChapStick and then continue your chat.

✚ Respiratory droplets are the most efficient mode of travel for germs. One sneeze or cough launches viruses and bacteria into the air, where they make contact with your eyes, nose, and mouth. Even if some germs don't directly meet their mark, they can live for up to 2 hours on surfaces like telephones, doorknobs, and keyboards.

4 *You receive a special-delivery package. The carrier arrives and offers his pen for you to sign the receipt. You:*

a. Don surgical gloves, sign the receipt, bring the package inside, and spray it with disinfectant before opening.

b. Sign the receipt, bring the package inside, and open it.

c. Chew on the pen while giving the receipt a once-over, sign it, and bring the package inside.

✚ Many of us don't think twice about using the common pens in public places like banks, doctor's offices, and restaurants—but they harbor colonies of germs. The simplest solution: Carry your own pen with you, and don't offer it to anyone else!

Does it work?

Antiviral medications such as Tamiflu

Worth a try (but only in certain situations)
For people who have H1N1 or seasonal flu, antivirals can shorten the duration of the illness by a day or two. "These medications are also being used for populations most at risk for complications— children, pregnant women, and adults with asthma or other medical conditions who have had a known exposure to H1N1. For them, antivirals can offer some protection," says Kathy J. Helzlsouer, MD, MHS, director of the prevention and research center at Mercy Medical Center in Baltimore. "However, because of the danger of viruses becoming resistant to these medications, not everyone should use them."

5 When should you wash your hands?

a. An easier question would be, when *shouldn't* I wash my hands?

b. Before eating and preparing meals and after using the bathroom, handling garbage, and touching animals.

c. Before meals . . . if I remember.

✚ Washing your hands is the easiest and most effective way to dramatically reduce your chances of getting sick. According to the Centers for Disease Control and Prevention, give your hands a good scrubbing before eating, handling medicine, and putting in contact lenses. Also lather up after using the bathroom and coming into contact with diapers, dirty objects (trash cans, cleaning rags, gardening tools), and bodily fluids like saliva and vomit. Of course, be

The Great Antibacterial Debate

In 2009, when concerns about the H1N1 virus were on the rise, one online retailer of cleaning products reported a 200 percent increase in its sales of hand sanitizers and liquid soaps. That's a lot of hand washing! But what's worrisome to some experts is the growing consumer reliance on antibacterial soaps and household cleaners to eliminate germs.

According to the Centers for Disease Control and Prevention, these products don't stop the spread of infection any better than the "regular" (nonantibacterial) variety. Not only that, but laboratory sure to wash before and after preparing food and tending to wounds.

KEY

If the majority of your answers are A: You are a Sanitizer. You take disinfecting to a level that even Mr. Clean would envy. Your vigilance is admirable, but take care not to overdo with antibacterial and antimicrobial products. Experts believe that they may bear some responsibility for the rise in "superbugs," pathogens that resist treatment. (To learn more, see "The Great Antibacterial Debate" below.)

If the majority of your answers are B: You are a Sentinel. You do your part not to spread germs by washing your hands frequently, covering your mouth when you sneeze or cough, and generally taking reasonable precautions to reduce your germ exposure. Hand sanitizers are your style, but surgical gloves and face masks? Not

studies have shown a link between antibacterial chemicals and drug-resistant bacteria.

And here's the real rub: Antibacterial products aren't even effective against viral infections like colds and flu, the very illnesses that cause us to load up on these products in the first place.

When it comes to clean hands—and good hygiene in general— it's the mechanics of washing rather than the ingredients in the soap that make the differ-ence. The simple action of rubbing your hands together loosens grime, while the soap binds to the germs and the water sends them down the drain.

So stick with regular soaps and household cleaners as much as possible. The exception is if someone in your home is elderly or ill or has a suppressed immune system. These populations are at high risk for infection; for them, using antibacteri-als can be beneficial.

so much. You can reinforce your efforts by taking advantage of the immune-boosting strategies in Chapter 5.

If the majority of your answers are C: You are a Spreader. You fear no germ, which is a good thing. But if you've noticed people ducking for cover when you're about to sneeze or cough, you may want to cultivate some healthier habits. Chapter 4 might be a good place to start.

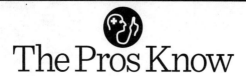

The Pros Know

Jill Benson
Flight attendant for United Airlines

Between the recirculated air, the tight quarters, and the shared seats and trays, airplanes are among the most germ-laden public places. The occasional flight for business or pleasure is one thing, but flight attendants like Jill Benson are exposed to all manner of microbes while they're on the job. Here's what she does to protect herself.

There is only so much that you can do to avoid germs, but I believe that every little action helps.

First and foremost, I constantly wash my hands. Some flight attendants I know wear light rubber gloves during the food and beverage service and when picking up trash. I use gloves, too, but usually only when I am helping someone who is sick. When I pick up empty cups, I never touch the rims. Some passengers do use face masks during the flight, which may help protect all of us.

Besides avoiding viruses and bacteria as much as possible, I do my best to take care of myself. I try to get plenty of sleep, eat healthfully, and exercise regularly. Although I feel like I should be doing more to protect myself, for the most part, these measures seem to work.

WHERE THE BUGS ARE

*A GERM'S-EYE VIEW OF
ITS FAVORITE PLACES*

Microbes and celebrities have at least one thing in common: Only the ones that behave badly seem to make headlines.

The vast majority of bacteria, viruses, and other microscopic bugs either show little interest in us humans or actually work to our advantage. Take, for instance, the 400 or so species of bacteria that

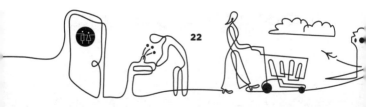

reside in your gut, writes microbiologist Anne Maczulak, PhD, in her book *The Five-Second Rule*. Without them, you couldn't digest food, synthesize vitamins, or manufacture proteins.

"Germs have been around us forever. There are a few precautions, but to live in constant fear is silly," Dr. Maczulak says. "The good microorganisms far outnumber the dangerous ones. That's something people don't always realize. They think all germs are bad."

Rather than trying to eliminate all microbes—which, besides being impossible, would backfire in the long run—it's best to marshal your resources against the harmful germs that tend to inhabit particular environments. In this chapter, we'll take a look around 12 common microbial hot spots (including your home) and offer some sensible strategies for outsmarting the not-so-friendly bugs that may be lurking there.

1. Public restrooms

For most of us, public restrooms rank highest on the ick scale. They aren't always the cleanest places—and that's judging by what we can see. As far as what we *can't* see ... well, we'd probably rather not know the details.

Interestingly, men's rooms tend to be slightly tidier than women's. Both, though, harbor bacteria on virtually every surface—including faucets and door handles, according to Dr. Maczulak. And by bacteria, she means the kind found in feces. (Presumably, viruses are widespread, too, but they're harder to measure.)

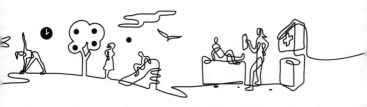

The Strategy

Move along. Overflowing trash cans and offensive smells suggest that the restroom hasn't been cleaned in a while. If your need isn't urgent, consider seeking another restroom, recommends Ruth Carrico, PhD, an assistant professor at the University of Louisville in Kentucky who specializes in disease prevention.

Don't fret about the toilet seat. Go ahead and line the toilet seat with toilet paper, or use one of those sanitary seat covers. It might protect you somewhat, Dr. Maczulak says. But studies suggest that toilet seats are relatively germ-free compared to other surfaces that a stream of people touch with their soiled hands.

Keep your purse aloft. Hang your purse from the hook on the stall door, Dr. Maczulak advises. If you put it on the floor, it's going to collect germs—and then you set your purse on the kitchen table or countertop when you get home.

Use your shoe. If the toilet doesn't flush automatically, and you're agile enough to reach the handle with your foot, flush that way, Dr. Carrico recommends. The fewer objects you touch with your hand, the better.

Wash your hands. In a study conducted on a university campus, 61 percent of women washed their hands with soap, compared to 37 percent of men. When the researchers put up a sign reminding of the importance of hand washing, nearly all the women scrubbed up. The men weren't so convinced; the percentage of male hand washers stayed about the same.

You should wash your hands after every expedition into a restroom. If you need pointers on how to wash well, see page 28.

Take a towel or two. If paper towels are available, use one to dry your hands, then turn off the faucet with it. Also use toweling to pull open the restroom door. Cover your hand with the paper towel to open the door, then prop the door with your foot and toss the towel into the trash can. For a door that pushes outward, nudge it open with your hip rather than grabbing the handle.

Changing a diaper? Clean up before and after. If you need to change a baby's diaper on a fold-down table in the restroom, clean it off first, Dr. Carrico suggests. You don't have to use a bleach wipe; baby wipes will do the trick, or use a paper towel that's dampened with water and a little soap. When you're done, clean the table one more time.

2. Restaurant buffets

With its endless array of food choices—entrées and sides, soups and salad fixings, breads and desserts, and assorted other offerings—a restaurant buffet has something for everyone. And microbes are waiting in line with the rest of us to dig in.

Buffet preparation is labor-intensive, which means that workers may not always wear gloves when handling food. And it may sit for hours on the buffet, where keeping hot and cold foods at their proper temperatures can be difficult.

But what makes buffets especially prime real estate for bacteria and viruses is the stream of coughing, scratching restaurant patrons who are putting their possibly dirty hands near or on the food, says Angela Fraser, PhD, an associate professor at Clemson University in South Carolina who trains restaurant employees in food safety.

The Strategy

Check for cleanliness. If the dining area looks unappetizing, can you imagine what the kitchen looks like? "If the owners really care about safety, they'll keep the dining area and buffet area clean," Dr. Fraser says.

Watch for quick turnaround. Food shouldn't sit on a buffet for more than 4 hours at a stretch, cautions Dr. Fraser, who teaches restaurant workers to use smaller serving dishes and replenish them more often. If you're in a restaurant with few other patrons and you see mounds of food on the buffet, that's a sign that it may have been out for too long.

While you're waiting to order, take notice of how often the staff replenishes the buffet. If the answer is not very often, then you might want to choose something from the menu.

Wait for replacements. Avoid spooning out the last remnants from a serving dish. Wait until a server returns with the fresh stuff.

Look for heat. Food that's served hot needs to be at least 135°F to resist microbial growth. At this temperature, food may produce steam, and though it won't burn your mouth, you might need to blow on it before taking a bite. If your soup or other normally hot item doesn't pass this test, consider helping yourself to something else.

Look for a sign. Patrons should use a fresh plate for each trip to the buffet, and the restaurant should post a sign that says so, Dr. Fraser says. "I really don't eat at places that don't have signs saying that children under 12 need to be accompanied by adults," Dr. Fraser adds. "I've seen children exhibit many bad behaviors at the buffet."

Tell the manager. Dr. Fraser has also spotted

ill-mannered adults nibbling a cherry tomato and then putting the rest back in the serving dish, or dipping a finger into the salad dressing. If you spot such behavior, alert a manager. A good restaurant will replace items that have been handled inappropriately, she says.

Wash your hands before you eat. Think about all the people who've handled the ladles, forks, and tongs before you. They may have blown their noses or visited the restroom, then headed for the buffet without bothering to wash their hands. You can't do much about their habits, but you can protect yourself. After you load up your plate, set it on your table and go wash *your* hands, Dr. Fraser advises. You'll scrub away any germs that others may have left on the buffet utensils.

3. Supermarkets

Singles aren't the only ones patrolling the produce aisle for hookups. Germs like to hang out in the supermarket, too.

Just think of the hundreds of shoppers that pass through each day, touching shopping cart handles, handling raw meat and produce, pulling items off shelves, and then putting them back. They're leaving behind a trail of microbes just waiting to hitch a ride on you.

The Strategy

Clean the shopping-cart handle. For a 2005 study, researchers sampled surfaces in more than 1,000 stores, gyms, theaters, and other public venues. Shopping-cart handles fared worse on several measures of yuckiness than elevator buttons, public telephones, and ink pens left out for public use.

Many stores now offer sanitizing wipes near the cart corral. It's probably a good idea to swipe one of these across your cart handle before you begin shopping, Dr. Fraser says. "I don't know how much it reduces the number of organisms, but it can't hurt," she adds.

Bag and bag again. Most supermarkets have plastic-bag dispensers all over the produce aisle, and maybe at the meat counter, too. Use them for your produce and meat purchases. Bagging keeps the produce from picking up germs from the cart, and the meat from dripping microbes onto other items in your cart. In fact, double-bagging these items might be wise, Dr. Fraser says.

Hand Washing How-Tos

You've been washing your hands since you were a little kid. Do you really need a tutorial? Probably. Keeping your hands clean is one of the most important steps you can take to avoid getting sick and spreading germs to other people.

No soap and water around? Use an alcohol-based hand sanitizer instead. They are fast acting and can significantly reduce the number of germs on your skin.

When you use soap and water:

✚ Wet your hands with clean running water—warm, if possible. Apply soap.

✚ Rub your hands together to make a lather. Scrub all surfaces and under your fingernails.

Mind your supermarket manners. Although everyone likes to get the most unblemished fruits and vegetables, try to limit the number of times you handle produce. It's just another opportunity to pick up germs—or pass them to someone else.

Skip the samples. Those bite-size morsels may be tempting, but you're better off taking a pass, Dr. Maczulak says. That goes doubly if you don't know how the food was prepared or how long it's been setting out.

Wash up. Once you're home, wash your hands before you start putting away your groceries, Dr. Fraser suggests. You'll get rid of any uninvited

✚ Continue rubbing your hands for 20 seconds. To keep track of the time, imagine singing "Happy Birthday" twice through.

✚ Rinse your hands thoroughly under running water.

✚ Dry your hands using a paper towel—yes, even at home. If you prefer to use hand towels from your bath, be sure to launder them regularly. (In a public restroom, you can use the air dryer if paper towels aren't available.)

When you use an alcohol-based hand sanitizer:

✚ Apply the product to the palm of one hand.

✚ Rub the palms of both hands together.

✚ Rub the product over all of the surfaces of your hands and fingers until your hands are dry.

guests of the microbial kind before they have a chance to settle in for an extended stay.

Clean your produce. The US Food and Drug Administration recommends thoroughly washing fruits and vegetables before eating them, even if you're going to peel them first. After washing your hands, rinse any fruits and veggies under cold running water. If they're small like berries or grapes, put them in a colander and gently tumble them under the water. If they're firm enough to take a little more handling, like cucumbers or apples, scrub them with a vegetable brush, too.

Drying your fruits and veggies with a paper

Does Your Child's Daycare Pass the Test?

Day care centers can't totally stop germs from coming through their doors, but they can take steps to reduce the spread, says Laura Jana, MD, a pediatrician in Omaha, Nebraska, and a member of the executive committee for early education and childcare for the American Academy of Pediatrics. Consider whether your child's daycare has implemented these germ-proofing practices; if not, you can be proactive in encouraging such practices—or at least take extra precautions to protect your child from infection.[all source 12 from chapter 7]

✚ Are parents given a "sick policy" explaining when kids should be kept at home?

✚ Are children sent home when they have a fever or diarrhea or they're vomiting?

towel may remove even more germs. But don't bother using soap or store-bought produce-cleaning products, the FDA advises.

4. Hotels

You've heard the expression "You get what you pay for." It might be right on the money, so to speak, when it's referring to the relative germiness of hotel rooms.

Charles P. Gerba, PhD, professor of soil, water, and environmental science at the University of Arizona in Tucson, says that in general, pricier rooms tend to be cleaner. "One of our studies

✚ Are children encouraged to wash their hands, especially before and after eating and after using the bathroom?

✚ Do staff members wash their hands regularly, especially before and after feeding children and after changing diapers and wiping noses?

✚ Do staff members wear gloves when changing diapers?

✚ If hand sanitizer is available, is it safely stored away from small children who might ingest it?

✚ Does the day care center use its own utensils and cups? (It's more sanitary if parents don't bring them from home, Dr. Jana says.)

✚ Is there a cleaning policy in place—for example, for sanitizing changing pads, toys, and desks?

✚ Does an outside cleaning service do deep cleaning? (They tend to do a better job, Dr. Jana says.)

✚ Are staff members required to get seasonal flu and H1N1 vaccines every year?

found that if you paid more than $50 a night, there was a much greater chance that the room was regularly disinfected. Rooms under $50 weren't."

Other, nonscientific research has found that germs abound no matter what the room rate. One media investigation found traces of urine or semen on bedspreads, chairs, walls, and floors. In another, hotel housekeepers rinsed drinking glasses with water or industrial cleaner, then used towels from the previous guests to dry them. Some staffers wore the same pair of latex gloves to clean the toilet and the glasses.

Although it's true that these investigations might not stand up to scientific scrutiny or represent widespread industry practices, they still beg the question: Just how clean is your hotel room?

The Strategy

Use disinfectant wipes. Clean the often-touched surfaces of your room, like door handles, light switches, faucets, telephones, and television remotes. If your room has a kitchenette, clean that, too.

Slip on flip-flops. Athlete's foot fungus can linger in bathrooms. Protect your feet by keeping them in disinfectable flip-flops whenever you use the bathroom—and if you visit the hotel pool, too.

Look for triple sheeting. Along with the usual bottom sheet, some hotels use two top sheets to sandwich the heavier bedding, like blankets and comforters. Wouldn't you rather sleep between easily laundered sheets than under a blanket that's harder to wash? (You could ask the housekeeping staff for an extra set of sheets, if you're up for triple-sheeting the bed yourself.)

And while we're on the subject ...

Remove the bedspread. It probably isn't laundered between guests' visits.

BYO glasses. As we've seen, the drinking glasses provided by a hotel may be less than sanitary, so pack your own plastic cups. And don't forget to use them!

5. Airplanes

Any mode of public transportation can be a breeding ground for microbes. In the case of air travel, though, the cramped quarters provide an especially welcoming environment for germs to multiply and spread, says Syed A. Sattar, PhD, professor emeritus of microbiology and director of the Centre for Research on Environmental Microbiology at the University of Ottawa in Ontario.

"It's not unusual for air travelers to cough, sneeze, or worse, vomit. Then other passengers inhale those germs or touch them on shared surfaces," Dr. Sattar explains. Plus, the stress of air travel may increase the chances of picking up a new infection or triggering an existing one.

Avoiding germs on international flights is even harder. "When people from all over the world crowd together in a confined space for hours at a time, you're going to be surrounded by all sorts of germs," Dr. Sattar says. "Some passengers may be moving back and forth from parts of the world where certain diseases are widespread."

And don't count on an airplane cabin being sanitized before you board. It's hard to know how often aircraft are cleaned, says Elizabeth Scott, PhD, codirector of the Simmons Center for Hygiene and

Health in Home and Community, and director of the Program in Public Health at Simmons College in Boston. But on 24-hour flights, they aren't cleaned at all.

The Strategy

Keep your bags off the floor. Store any carry-on luggage in the overhead compartment. You'll need to stow your purse or briefcase for takeoff, but once you're free to move around, move your bag to your seat.

Disinfect nearby surfaces. Keep disinfectant wipes in your purse or briefcase. Use them to clean your tray table, the armrest, headphones—anything you touch.

Stay hydrated. A study published in the *Journal of Environmental Health Research* found that dry airplane air increases your chances of getting the sniffles. A thin layer of mucus in your nose and throat normally flushes out bacteria and viruses. If the air is dry, this lining dries out, too—and you're more vulnerable to infection.

Be wary of bathrooms. Airplane restrooms are tiny, cramped, and used frequently, Dr. Gerba notes. "On any given flight, 50 people may use the same toilet—75 if it's a discount airline," he says.

If you gotta go, be sure to wash your hands with soap and water once you've finished your business. Then use a paper towel to turn off the water and open the door. As an extra precaution, you may want to use a hand sanitizer before you get back to your seat.

Ask to be reseated. If you're sitting near a coughing or sneezing passenger, ask the flight attendant if you can move. If another seat is available, or if someone is willing to switch with you, the attendant may be able to accommodate you.

6. Hospitals

You probably think of hospitals as places to get well. And they are—usually. But sometimes they can make you sick.

"Any infection you can catch outside the hospital you can catch inside, too," Dr. Gerba says. Among the most worrisome hospital-acquired infections: staph (*Staphylococcus aureus*), MRSA (methicillin-resistant *Staphylococcus aureus*), and *Clostridium difficile.*

Staph infections cause a red, pimple-like rash that usually responds to antibiotics. If it doesn't, it may be MRSA—which, incidentally, can appear in otherwise healthy people. *C. difficile* are fecal

Does it work?

Astragalus

Don't bother

"There really are no good data on astragalus," says Margaret Lewin, MD, clinical assistant professor of medicine at Cornell University and chief medical director of Cinergy Health. Also, much like medications such as aspirin and beta-blockers, astragalus gets circulated throughout the body and therefore could cause unwanted side effects.

"I'm really concerned about mucking around with the immune system with immunostimulants and immunomodulators," Dr. Lewin says. "I would be wary of astragalus, especially if you have any kind of immune deficiency."

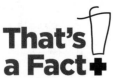

That's a Fact

A dry mouth is a welcome mat for germs. "Saliva does two things to protect you against illness: It provides a sticky place to trap viruses and bacteria, and it contains germ-fighting antibodies," says Margaret Lewin, MD, clinical assistant professor of medicine at Cornell University and chief medical director of Cinergy Health. You can wash away potential illnesses with lots of hydrating fluids, she says.

bacteria. They cause diarrhea as well as more serious conditions such as colitis and sepsis, which spreads through the bloodstream.

Health-care workers can transmit any of these bacteria by touching surfaces or handling items with unwashed hands. If you touch the same surfaces or items, you can become infected, too.

The Strategy

Get a flu vaccine. It's the best way to avoid the flu, which is known to raise the risk of certain kinds of staph infection.

Wash your hands—and remind others to do the same. Whether you're a visitor or a patient, you can help stop the spread of bacteria and other germs by washing your hands with soap and water or using an alcohol-based hand sanitizer. And watch to be sure that health-care workers are scrubbing up, too—even if they wear gloves when providing care.

Watch where you put your hands. Doorknobs, television remotes, bed rails, toilets—any surface that people touch can become a repository for bugs. Ideally, these surfaces are disinfected daily. But it's best to be cautious and limit your contact with them as much as possible.

7. Workplaces

These days, many of us spend so much time on the job that we view our colleagues as an extended family. We share everything with each other—including more than a few germs.

"Disease transmission is more frequent when many people are indoors together in a confined space," Dr. Sattar observes. "I call air the environmental equalizer. You may not drink the water in your workplace, and you may not eat the food. But you have to breathe the same air as everyone else." And if that air is heavily contaminated with disease-causing germs, infections will spread more easily.

The Strategy

Don't eat at your desk. You might save time by multitasking, but you're also increasing your chances of getting sick. Every object in your workspace—your phone, your keyboard, your stapler, your pen—is a potential hangout for germs. "One study found 400 times more germs on an average desktop than on a toilet seat," Dr. Gerba says.

Disinfect. Use disinfectant wipes to clean any shared supplies and equipment, such as telephones, fax machines, printers, and photocopiers.

Keep your hands to yourself. Try to avoid shaking hands during cold and flu season. If you must, be sure to wash your hands or use hand sanitizer as soon as you can afterward.

Clean up before heading home. If you keep a water bottle or coffee cup at your desk, empty and wash it at the end of each workday. And of course, don't share cups or bottles with anyone else.

Maintain your distance. Avoid close contact

with anyone who has a cold or flu. And if you get sick, by all means stay home.

8. Gyms

We go to the gym to get fit, right? So it's hard to imagine that we might come home with more than our gym bags and water bottles. But shared surfaces in gyms—not to mention their locker rooms—are perfect environments for germs to flourish.

"Staph and MRSA thrive in hot, sweaty places," Dr. Gerba says. "They tend to lurk around where people wear the same gym clothes and use the same towels for several days or several workouts."

The fungus that causes athlete's foot also loves showers and locker rooms, Dr. Sattar says. "When people already contaminated with the fungus walk barefoot on these warm, damp surfaces, it's quite easy for the fungus to spread to others who are also walking barefoot."

Many gyms try to head off the spread of infection by providing spray bottles near workout stations and pieces of equipment. "Gym managers suggest that you spray the equipment after you use it, but it's not clear what products are being used, if everyone uses them, or if they're effective," Dr. Scott says.

The Strategy

Be nosy. Ask the gym staff what kind of disinfectant they use and how they know it's working. If you don't like the answer, ask if you can bring your own instead.

Carry sanitizer with you. When you grasp

handrails or barbells, you're also grasping all of the microbial crud that the people before you left behind. So it's a good idea to clean your hands with sanitizer every time you change equipment.

Practice downward dog safely. Who knows whether your yoga studio disinfects the mats they use? You're better off investing in your own. Be sure to keep it clean by washing and disinfecting according to the manufacturer's instructions.

Skip the bare feet. When you're in the locker room, wear flip-flops at all times, including in the shower.

Use a bandage if necessary. If you have any cuts or scrapes, keep them covered while you're working out.

9. Day Care and Schools

Like peanut butter and jelly, day-care centers and germs just seem to go together. In fact, several of our experts describe these facilities as "pits of disease."

Children of all ages are in day care, with the youngest often still in diapers. This makes cleanliness a real concern. "If diaper-changing areas aren't kept meticulously clean and separate from the rest of the facility, germs can be transmitted," Dr. Scott says. "That's especially true if the staff doesn't practice good hand hygiene."

What's worse, toddlers love to put things into their mouths; it's how they make sense of their world. Older kids often transmit germs by touching their own faces. "Studies show that they may touch their faces 81 times an hour," Dr. Gerba says.

Many of the same germs found in day-care

centers—especially rotovirus and norovirus, both of which cause digestive symptoms—can circulate around elementary, middle, and high schools, too. MRSA is becoming a big concern for scholastic athletic facilities, as the bacteria can linger on surfaces such as barbells and mats.

The Strategy

Teach good hand hygiene. Encourage kids to wash their hands with soap and water for 20 seconds, and to repeat many times a day. For extra protection, they can use alcohol-based hand sanitizer. A study of 285 elementary-school students found that kids were less likely to miss school because of gastrointestinal illness if they used sanitizers and if their desks were disinfected daily, Dr. Gerba says.

Hit the shower. Because MRSA can spread through skin-to-skin contact, student athletes should take showers with soap and water after wrestling matches and all other athletic events or practices.

Stay on schedule. Be sure that your child's recommended vaccinations are up-to-date.

Skip school when necessary. When kids get sick, they should be kept home from school or day care until they've been fever free for at least 24 hours.

10. Play areas

Kids almost assuredly look at a play area and see nothing but opportunities for fun. As the grownup, you need to see it for what it really is: a place for germs to congregate.

The Strategy

Watch their hands. Occasionally remind kids to keep their fingers out of their mouths and noses and away from their faces in general. (Remember, the face presents many different pathways into the body.) If you see a wayward finger probing around, tell your kid to stop.

Keep an eye on playmates, too. If you see other children who are coughing, wiping runny noses, or showing other signs of an illness that could be passed along, gently steer your kid to a different area, Dr. Carrico suggests.

Be prudent when poolside. Fecal matter can find its way into the water, causing swimmers to fall ill. Several disease outbreaks associated with water parks have been reported to the Centers for Disease Control and Prevention; even more may have gone unreported.

Stress to your kids that they need to keep the water out of their mouths whenever they go swimming. Make sure that they wash their hands after they get out of the water, especially if they're going to eat.

The CDC advises parents to bathe their kids—particularly their kids' bottoms—before going swimming. And if a child has diarrhea, be polite and keep him or her out of the water altogether.

Show your zoo savvy. Petting zoos are popular, but kids may be putting their hands on more critters than you'd care to imagine: Many disease outbreaks related to *Escherichia coli* have been linked to petting zoos and similar venues.

When you visit any attraction that allows children to interact with animals, leave food, drinks, strollers, baby bottles, and pacifiers outside the area. Stay away from any animals that look sick, and remind kids not to touch their faces until their hands are clean.

Work up a lather. Once you leave a play area, have your kids wash their hands with soap and water. If none are available, then use an alcohol-based hand sanitizer instead. Keep in mind that when the weather turns colder, a kid's hands can get dry and chapped just like a grown-up's—and putting sanitizer on broken skin can really hurt. You can protect your child's skin by applying lotion or moisturizer as needed.

11. Dorms

For the average college student, housekeeping ranks low on the list of priorities—somewhere between "skip party to study for test" and "start researching term paper due 4 months from now." But your college-bound teen or twenty-something could benefit from a lesson in dorm-room hygiene.

As Dr. Scott notes, most colleges leave dorm-room cleaning to the students—and they aren't always savvy about what a thorough cleaning entails. But a tidy room, combined with good personal hygiene, can help them to stay healthy during what can be a very stressful time.

College campuses pose many of the same health risks as lower-grade schools, in terms of infectious illness. "At college, though, students live in close quarters with each other, and they spend their days in one crowded classroom after another," Dr. Scott says.

One illness that can hit college campuses especially hard is bacterial meningitis, or meningococcal disease. It's an inflammation of the membranes that cover the brain and spinal cord, causing high fever, headache, stiff neck, nausea, and vomiting. Dorm-dwelling college freshmen are at particular risk for infection, which is why it's recommended that they get a meningococcal vaccine before heading off to college.

The Strategy

Clean up before moving in. Things can be hectic on moving day, but if time permits, you should give your kid's dorm room a thorough cleaning and disinfecting to clear out any lingering germs.

Target surfaces. Give your college student a supply of disinfectant wipes and encourage him or her to do at least a surface cleaning on a regular basis. Pay particular attention to any area that comes into contact with food, such as a microwave or refrigerator, as well as shared surfaces such as desktops and computer keyboards and mice.

Make some suds. College students will wash clothes without laundry detergent to save a few pennies. But they really need the soap in order to get rid of odor, soil, dirt, and bacteria.

Strip the bed. Bedding and towels should be washed in hot water at least weekly. The high temperature helps remove germs from fabrics.

Avoid mold and mildew. Wet or damp laundry should be hung on a drying rack. Putting it away before it's dry can invite mildew and mold.

Slip on flip-flops. Asking college students to wear flip-flops isn't too big of a stretch. A nonslip pair is good for protecting feet from the fungi that inhabit dorm bathrooms and showers.

Scrub up. By now it goes without saying that washing hands well can go a long way toward keeping germs at bay. Soap and water are best, but when they aren't handy, an alcohol-based hand sanitizer will do.

Pamper your immune system. Late nights and pizza runs are college traditions, but both can punish the body's natural defenses if they become habits. Gently remind your college student to get plenty of rest and eat lots of immune-boosting fruits and vegetables, both of which will fortify his or her disease resistance.

12. Your Home

Though they don't help pay the rent or mortgage, hordes of bacteria and viruses may be living quite comfortably under your roof. Even keeping your home spotless might not be enough to evict these unwelcome guests, unless you know precisely where they might be hunkering down.

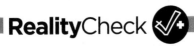

*Reality*Check

Colds and flu are most contagious before symptoms appear.

"Not necessarily true," says Erika Schwartz, MD, chief medical officer of www.healthandprevention. com. You may be contagious before symptoms set in, but you aren't necessarily *most* contagious then.

Usually you know when you're coming down with something. Those early symptoms— fatigue, sore throat, general malaise—should be your cue to take extra-good care of yourself by eating well and getting plenty of rest.

"It's also the time to stay home," Dr. Schwartz says. "Too many people go to work and public places when they're sick. But by not toughing it out, you protect yourself and everyone around you."

The Strategy

De-germ your kitchen sink. Which would you rather eat from, your toilet or your kitchen sink? Neither is very appetizing, of course, but the average kitchen sink is home to 1,000 times more bacteria than the average toilet. It isn't all that surprising, when you consider the bits of food that swirl around and down the drain, not to mention the gunk in that stinky pit known as the garbage disposal.

According to Dr. Fraser, the sink is one of two spots in the kitchen that she cleans "religiously." She pours a teakettle of boiling water over the entire sink surface and down both drains to kill germs and get rid of the drain odors. You can do this yourself, but be sure that your drainpipes can handle the hot water. As an alternative, mix 1 tablespoon of bleach (or a capful from the bleach jug) into a gallon of water and clean the sink and drains with this solution.

The other must-clean spot is the refrigerator, where old food and crusty spills can feed germs. Once a week, Dr. Fraser tosses out any leftovers and gives the shelves and other surfaces a wipe-down—first with soap and water, then with diluted bleach.

Sanitize your sponge. If you use a sponge to clean off countertops and other kitchen surfaces, it soaks up a lot of potentially nasty germs. You should clean it regularly so that you aren't smearing its microbial contents all over the rest of your kitchen. To do this, simply dampen the sponge and then microwave it for a minute, or run it through the dishwasher on the drying cycle.

Keep a clean carpet machine. When you run the vacuum, it sucks in bacteria along with food for those bacteria, so the germs can continue to thrive in the vacuum bag. Use antibacterial bags if they're available for your vacuum model, and replace them regularly. Change the bag outdoors, so the inevitable cloud of debris won't infiltrate the rest of your home.

Take off your shoes. The world is a dirty place, and you can step into all kinds of foul material as you go about your business. Why track the germ-laden remnants of the day into your home? Leave your shoes by the door instead.

Turn up the heat on laundry. Dirty clothing may be dirtier than you think. Dr. Gerba has written at length in scientific journals about how much fecal matter is in an average adult's worn underwear (one-tenth of a gram, the equivalent of one-quarter of a peanut), and how many nasty bacteria and viruses can survive in cold or warm water. (It's quite a few, since if you start with 100 million bacteria and reduce them by 99 percent, you still have a million left.)

The take-home message from several of Dr. Gerba's studies is to wash laundry in hot water whenever possible, use bleach in the washer if you can, and dry clothing on the hot setting. Even this won't kill all of the germs, but it'll help. Also, wash your hands after you transfer the laundry from the washer to the dryer.

The Pros Know

Kathy J. Helzlsouer, MD, MHS
*Director of the prevention and research
center at Mercy Medical Center in Baltimore*

Dr. Helzlsouer investigates how to prevent the spread of viruses and bacteria, and she practices what she preaches every day.

When I was in medical school, one of my professors came into class on the first day and said, "Colds are a psychosomatic illness." He then went on to explain the connection between mind and body and how periods of stress make us more vulnerable to getting sick. And it's true. There have been plenty of studies to show that people have a limited response to vaccines when they are under stress and an increased response to them when they are managing stress with relaxation techniques, sleep, and a healthy diet.

To manage my own stress, and thus to keep my immune system in the best shape possible, I get enough sleep, eat well, and practice deep breathing. I also wash my hands before and after I see a patient; I don't want to give them anything, and I don't want to get anything from them.

When something is circulating around the office, like a gastrointestinal virus, I clean all of the doorknobs down with disinfectant wipes. I am particularly careful when it comes to common touch areas. Anything that anyone has touched can become contaminated with what that person had on his or her hands. That's why you should always wash your hands.

CHAPTER

4

THE
IMMUNE
BUSTERS

*FORTIFY YOUR DEFENSES
AGAINST THIS DIRTY DOZEN*

More than anything else, your everyday habits can make or break your body's ability to
protect itself from the bug du jour. Andrew
Eisenberg, MD, a family physician and medical
advisor for the nonprofit group Families Fighting
Flu in Sarasota, Florida, says, "I've been around
people who are very ill, including with the swine
flu, and I have not gotten sick. I'm convinced

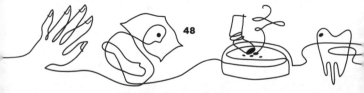

48

that my behaviors are helping to protect me from infection."

The things you do—or don't do—in the course of your daily routine can weaken your immune system, leading to more frequent colds or infections, or just a general sense of *blah*. The good news is, by dropping the bad habits, you have that many more ways to strengthen your defenses and avoid sickness.

Touching Your Face and Biting Your Nails

Of all the germ carriers that we routinely encounter, two of the worst offenders are literally at arm's length. "We all have a tendency to put our hands in places they really shouldn't go," Dr. Eisenberg says. "We don't realize the volume of bacteria we pick up, simply because we can't see them." And we touch our faces incredibly often: A study from the University of California, Berkeley, found that we make contact with our noses, eyes, or lips an average of once every 4 minutes.

Why it's bad Carrying around literally handfuls of germs means that habitually touching your face is an easy way to deliver a dose of virus or bacteria right to where it can settle in and make you sick. "The portals of entry are all right there," Dr. Eisenberg says. "In fact, the main paths of influenza transmission are through the eyes and the nose."

Make it better Scratching or picking your nose is a habit to drop right away, as is rubbing your eyes or pulling on your eyelids or eyelashes. Nail or cuticle biting is also a problem, not only because

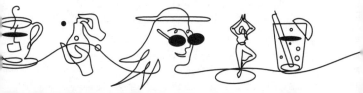

That's a Fact

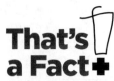

To maintain personal hygiene, you should respect personal space.

Many viruses and bacteria are transmitted via saliva droplets, which can travel a good few feet when propelled by a cough or sneeze. A good rule of thumb is to allow at least 3 feet between yourself and someone else. "With H1N1, the recommendation is to stand back as much as 6 feet," says recently retired emergency-room physician Kathleen Handal, MD, author of *The American Red Cross First Aid & Safety Handbook* and president of www.dochandal.com.

you're introducing germs into your mouth but also because you're constantly bringing your hands up to your face, potentially spreading bacteria near your eyes and nose in the process.

To train yourself to keep your hands below chin height, try this mildly painful trick: Wear a rubber band around your wrist and snap it against your inner wrist every time you catch yourself touching your face. It's a form of negative feedback that will discourage you from picking, poking, and otherwise pawing at your facial parts.

To break a nail-biting habit, the Mayo Clinic recommends regular manicuring, clipping nails short and filing them smooth. You can also try wearing a special bitter-tasting polish to remind you not to put your fingers in your mouth.

If you just can't seem to keep your hands away from your face, the next best thing is to reduce the microbial load with frequent hand washing. The Centers for Disease Control and Prevention (CDC) recommends lathering up with soap and warm water for at least 20 seconds. Rinse your hands well, then dry with a paper towel or air dryer.

Not Getting Enough Sleep

The occasional bout of sleeplessness probably won't have any lasting impact on your immune system. But watch out for chronic insomnia or a serious sleep deficit, because these definitely can make you more likely to come down with whatever is going around. When you are trying not to get sick, more rest is best.

Why it's bad The science is clear: A lack of sleep undermines immune function. According to researchers at Carnegie Mellon University in Pittsburgh, people who got less than 7 hours of sleep were nearly three times more likely to come down with a cold than those who had 8 or more hours of shut-eye.

A study from the CDC found that only 1 in 3 Americans gets close to the 7 to 8 hours we generally need to function at our best. And a very tired 16 percent of adults get less than 6 hours per night, according to the National Sleep Foundation.

All this tossing and turning, and late-to-bed and early-to-rise activity, does not bode well for staying healthy. "Your nervous system is in parasympathetic mode during sleep," explains Simon Yu, MD, a board-certified internist in St. Louis, Missouri, who also practices complementary and alternative medicine. "If it doesn't get sufficient downtime to rejuvenate and repair, your immune function will suffer." The parasympathetic nerves regulate your internal organs, including your heart, and manage crucial functions such as digestion and elimination.

Make it better If you're finding that time is not on your side when it comes to getting enough sleep, try creating a bedtime ritual, just as you might have done when you were a kid. A good place to start is by lowering the lights and turning off your cell phone when you're getting ready to turn in. A study from Wayne State University in Detroit found that talking on a cell phone before going to bed caused a 13 percent drop in deep sleep, the kind that helps the body recover from daily wear and tear.

You might also try taking a warm shower about an hour before hitting the hay. The warm water is relaxing, and more important, the drop in body temperature afterward will encourage a natural downshift to sleep.

Many sleep experts recommend keeping your bedroom cool, but not cold—between 54° and 75°F. This, too, turns down your body's thermostat, which encourages deeper sleep.

Smoking

It goes without saying that cigarette smoking is the granddaddy of all bad health habits. Everyone knows that smoking introduces toxins into the body,

RealityCheck ✔✓

Starve a fever, feed a cold.

There may be something to this popular proverb. Fever—defined as a core body temperature of 100.4°F or higher—is a sign that your body is fending off an invading virus or bacteria. At this critical time in the healing process, you don't want your body to redirect its resources to digestion, as it would need to do if you're eating solid foods. Sticking with a liquid diet during a fever is easier on your digestive tract, and it helps maintain your body's fluid balance.

but you might be surprised to learn exactly how it increases your risk of respiratory infection and flu.

Why it's bad Cigarettes are the perfect way to become an ideal host for bacteria and viruses, says Ann Carey Tobin, MD, an integrative medicine specialist in private practice in Delmar, New York. Smoking weakens cilia, the tiny projections on lung cells that work to move debris and secretions out and away from the lungs. It also damages the protective bacteria that normally hold the line against unfriendly germs inside the lungs.

When smokers catch a respiratory ailment, they are much more likely to get bacterial infections, Dr. Tobin says. That's because of their reduced ability to fend off an invading bug.

Make it better There's really only one way to avoid smoking's insidious effects, and that's to quit. You've got plenty of help, from medications like Chantix and Zyban to online quit programs and support groups (check out the American Lung Association's free program at www.ffsonline.org). And don't forget about nicotine gum and patches.

Fear of—or Overzealous—Flossing

The plaque that forms on teeth and sets the stage for gum disease contains as many as 400 different bacterial species. The best and easiest way to get rid of them is by flossing regularly and properly. That's something many of us don't do.

Why it's bad When we don't floss, we invite bacterial infection and gum disease, a serious medical condition that can lead to tooth loss, among other problems. Researchers at Columbia University

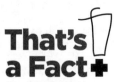

That's a Fact

in New York City believe that the chronic inflammation associated with gum disease stresses the immune system, opening the door to other infections.

Just as not flossing can lead to trouble, so can flossing too furiously, Dr. Yu says. Vigorous flossing that injures the gums can spread bacteria into the bloodstream. This condition, called bacteremia, can be responsible for systemic infections that cause fever, aches, and pains.

Make it better Done gently and correctly, flossing shouldn't hurt. Try to avoid snapping the strand down into your gum; instead imagine that you're carefully buffing the sides of each tooth with the floss.

If you're still having trouble, the next time you visit your dentist, ask your hygienist to teach you proper flossing technique. You might also ask which type of floss you should be using. There are lots to choose from, and one may work better for you than others.

For those who are new to flossing or who have limited hand dexterity, the Academy of General Dentistry recommends a prethreaded flosser or floss holder. They look like miniature hacksaws and are available in the dental care aisle of just about any drugstore.

If your gums bleed when you floss, you may already have gum disease. Other signs include red or tender gums and a gum line that seems to pull away from your teeth. See your dentist as soon as possible for treatment that will protect your teeth and your overall health.

Consuming Too Much Caffeine

Caffeine is the active ingredient in two of the most popular drinks in the world: coffee and tea. Although many studies now show that caffeine has measurable health benefits, including antioxidant properties, in this case more of a good thing is not necessarily better.

Why it's bad Caffeine depletes the body's stores of zinc, according to Lauri Grossman, DC, a licensed chiropractor and chair of the department of medicine and humanistic studies at the American Medical College of Homeopathy in New York City. "Zinc is a mineral that is necessary for healing," Dr. Grossman says. "If someone has a cold, it is much more likely to lead to a serious illness such as the flu if the person's zinc supply is low."

Make it better You don't need to give up caffeine entirely. Most studies show negligible negative effects at less than 3 cups of coffee a day; that's 200 to 300 milligrams of caffeine total. Or you might try switching from coffee to tea, which has about half the caffeine of regular brewed coffee (and many proven health benefits besides).

If you're committed to giving up caffeine altogether, be sure to taper off over a few weeks to avoid withdrawal headaches and fatigue. You can ease the transition with a "half-caf" blend (such as Green Mountain Roasters or Eight O'Clock brand) or just mix your own.

Not Washing Your Hands

A time-honored protective measure, hand washing is more important than ever when contagious bugs abound. When researchers analyzed the results of studies conducted over a span of 40 years, they found that improvements in hand hygiene have reduced respiratory-illness rates by more than 20 percent.

Still, relatively few of us actually wash our hands as often as we should. If you've gotten a little lazy about lathering up, you may want to reconsider.

Why it's bad When you don't wash up after touching potentially contaminated surfaces or items, you are unnecessarily exposing yourself to infection, Dr. Tobin says. "Washing your hands is not the only way to keep yourself safe, but it's definitely a big part of the formula."

Make it better The CDC still favors plain soap and water as the best for hand washing because it removes the most dirt and debris. But maybe you can't get to a sink when you really need one. For those occasions, Allison Aiello, PhD, professor of epidemiology at the University of Michigan in Ann Arbor, suggests investing in a bottle of waterless, alcohol-based hand sanitizer. Choose a gel or liquid product that contains at least 60 percent alcohol.

Breathing through Your Mouth

Habitually breathing through your mouth doesn't just leave you looking perpetually confused. It also increases your risk for respiratory illness.

Why it's bad About 20 percent of us are chronic mouth breathers, either as an acquired habit or because of asthma or structural problems with the nose, according to physiotherapist Brenda Stimpson, president of Breathingwise in Pasadena, California. Mouth breathers get more colds and flu in part because unlike the lungs, the mouth has no cilia to trap the fine particles that cause irritation. In addition, research shows that cells in the sinuses surrounding the nose produce nitric oxide, which helps to sanitize inhaled air. Air that comes in through your mouth misses out on these barriers, which gives microbes a straight shot to your lungs.

Make it better The best way to break a mouth-breathing habit is to force yourself to breathe through your nose. "It may be difficult at first, because you'll feel as though you aren't getting enough air," Stimpson says. "But over a few hours to a few days of consistent nose breathing, it should become free and clear."

Shunning the Sun

Most dermatologists will tell you to wear sunscreen every day. And that's pretty good advice, if your mission is to keep wrinkles at bay. Unfortunately, when you prevent the sun's UV rays from reaching your skin, you also interfere with your body's ability to synthesize its own supply of vitamin D.

Why it's bad As Dr. Tobin observes, vitamin D is very important to the health of your immune system. Studies are finding that vitamin D deficiency contributes to weakened immunity and increased susceptibility to flu, not to mention a greater risk for osteoporosis, depression, and even some cancers.

Make it better Very few foods contain vitamin D naturally; fish and fish liver oils are about the only good sources, and you'd need to consume quite a bit of both to obtain a meaningful amount of the vitamin. The best way to get your D is from the sun.

You needn't spend a lot of time soaking up the sun's rays; just 10 to 15 minutes of sun on unprotected skin should cover you. Try to go outside when the sun is least likely to burn—usually before 10 a.m. or after 4 p.m. If you intend to be outdoors for longer than the recommended time frame, then definitely slather on the sunscreen.

If you can't tolerate the sun, or if you live in a northern climate with limited sunlight, you might consider boosting your vitamin D intake with supplements. Current government guidelines recommend 200 to 600 IU daily, but many researchers believe that we need as much as 1,000 IU a day, if not more. You can always ask your doctor for a blood test to check your vitamin D status if you're unsure.

Overindulging a Sweet Tooth

It's perfectly fine to enjoy a thick piece of birthday cake or a box of chocolate-covered raisins at the movie theater ... once in a while. But if you eat sweets on a regular basis, you may unwittingly be rolling out the welcome mat for microbes.

Why it's bad A steady diet of sugary foods can prevent your white blood cells—your body's natural infection fighters—from effectively engulfing and destroying bacteria. It also causes unhealthy swings in blood glucose and insulin. "Even if you don't have diabetes, your body will wind up investing a lot of effort in maintaining homeostasis rather than patrolling for illness-causing invaders," Dr. Eisenberg says.

Make it better If you know you'll be having a high-sugar day, you can help steady your blood glucose levels by eating more soluble fiber, says Barbara Quinn, RD, author of *The Diabetes DTOUR Diet*. This form—found in beans, broccoli, and apples, among other foods—of fiber interferes with and slows down carbohydrate absorption in the intestines, which keeps blood sugar on an even keel.

Soda is a major source of sugar in the typical American diet. But you may want to think twice before trading your full-sugar sodas for the zero-calorie variety, which have been linked to metabolic syndrome and a higher risk of heart disease. Instead, try flavored seltzer, which has no calories or artificial sweeteners but provides soda-like fizz and flavor. Or try a sparkling juice, which you can water down with seltzer to reduce your sugar consumption even further.

Being a Worrywart

Trying not to worry is a lot like trying not to move for the next half hour—it's easier said than done. Goodness knows there's more than enough to fret about these days. Though you can't escape stress completely, you should try to keep it from getting the best of you. Otherwise, it can take a toll on your immune system, among many other aspects of your health.

Why it's bad When you're under stress, your adrenal glands release cortisol, a potent hormone that is useful in emergency situations but causes trouble over the long run. Chronically high cortisol—common in those who are anxiety prone or type A—challenges the body's ability to function normally, leading to a depressed immune response and increased vulnerability to infectious illness.

Make it better Stress can result from both positive and negative events in your life, says clinical psychologist Patricia Farrell, PhD. To get a sense of your current stress level, Dr. Farrell suggests doing an online search for the Holmes-Rahe scale and then taking the simple test. Your score may surprise you, but it also should motivate you to take control of the stressors in your life.

One of the easiest ways to improve your ability to handle stress is to exercise regularly. "We're not talking about pumping iron or even going to a gym," Dr. Farrell explains. "I tell my patients to walk in place if that is the only activity they can do. Just move your body."

Dr. Farrell also recommends regular bouts of laughter to protect your immune system against stress's effects. In several studies, people's cortisol levels dropped substantially in response to laughter.

Polluting Your Indoor Air

According to the Environmental Protection Agency, we Americans spend up to 90 percent of our time indoors. So maybe it shouldn't come as a surprise that the concentration of airborne pollutants is worse in our homes, schools, and workplaces than it is outside.

Why it's bad Indoor air can harbor pollen, mold, dust, pet dander, cigarette smoke, soot, and other substances that irritate your airways and lungs. "When your nose and eyes are moist and itchy, you become an ideal host for infection and an attractive site for bacteria to grow," Dr. Tobin explains.

Make it better Dr. Yu recommends installing an air filter in your home to remove air pollutants. Be sure to choose a unit with a true HEPA filter to safely remove 99 percent of airborne particles.

Also, be mindful of your indoor air space when cleaning or painting. Choose low- or zero-VOC paints, which have less vaporous chemicals in them. And opt for homemade cleaning products like a simple spray bottle of vinegar and water, which is good for wiping down just about any surface and smells fresh without artificial fragrance.

Attempting to eliminate or cover up bad air smells with scented fresheners only adds another layer of pollutants. "You're just masking a foul odor by introducing a stronger one," says James Sublett, MD, chief of pediatric allergy and immunology at the University of Louisville School of Medicine. To really clear the air, leave the scented sprays and other artificial air fresheners on the supermarket shelf and open a window instead.

Ignoring Your Need for Water
Water is the single most important nutrient for your body, and the most plentiful, accounting for 60 percent of your total weight. Allowing

yourself to get even a little bit dehydrated can undermine all of your body's systems, including your immune system.

Why it's bad As Dr. Grossman explains, not drinking enough water prevents your cells, tissues, and organs from operating at their best. It also impedes your body's ability to eliminate waste products generated by normal metabolism, stress, and illness. "All of the hand washing in the world won't get rid of the toxins that are on the inside," Dr. Grossman says.

Make it better If you just can't swallow plain old water, by all means try one of the new flavored varieties—but choose wisely. As a rule of thumb, you should steer clear of any water beverage that has a long ingredient list. Only buy brands with ingredients that you recognize.

You might try jazzing up a glass of tap or filtered water with an old-fashioned lemon slice, a fresh mint leaf, or some grated ginger. It's cheaper than a bottled beverage, and it's available wherever faucets are flowing.

The Pros Know

Sue DeCotiis, MD
*Board-certified internal medicine specialist
in private practice in New York City*

As an internist, Dr. DeCotiis knows how quickly and easily infections start and how frequently she's exposed to them as part of her job. Here's how she avoids becoming a patient herself.

First, I do all the obvious things—washing my hands often and wiping down surfaces like doorknobs, countertops, elevator buttons, and faucets. When I'm out and about, I carry paper towels and use them to grasp door handles and faucet handles, thus limiting my exposure to germs.

In my office, the examination tables are set so that patients are at a right angle to me. That way, when patients cough or sneeze, I don't get a face full of germs.

At home, I don't allow handbags or briefcases on tables, kitchen counters, or beds. These things have been on the floor of a bathroom stall or maybe even on the street, picking up all sorts of bacteria and viruses.

Especially during cold and flu season, I make sure to sleep at least 8 hours a night. If I feel tired, I realize that my body is trying to tell me something, and I hit the sack.

Beyond that, I eat lots of garlic in raw or pill form (cooked garlic is probably ineffective). There is no conclusive evidence that it eradicates colds or flu, but some research has shown that it may shorten the duration of a respiratory infection. (People on blood thinners should use garlic sparingly, however.)

5

THE IMMUNE BOOSTERS

50 WAYS TO LEAVE YOUR LYSOL (AND STAY DISEASE-FREE!)

Your body is capable of many amazing things, but perhaps none is as extraordinary as its ability to protect you from infection. Millions of cells, each with a highly specialized function, communicate and collaborate with each other not only to destroy pathogens but also to remember them should they try to invade again.

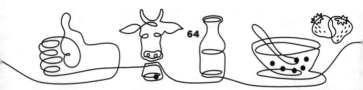

All this goes on without your even realizing it—well, except for the occasional microbe that slips through undetected. Given the sheer volume of germs that you encounter on a daily basis, your immune system's track record is quite impressive. But it needs proper care and feeding to keep on doing what it does so well.

That's where you come in. By taking steps to strengthen your immune function and reduce your germ exposure, you can greatly improve your odds of not getting sick. We're not asking you to reinvent your lifestyle for the sake of staying healthy, because you really don't need to. As you'll see in this chapter, sometimes the simplest changes can yield the most dramatic results.

With guidance from our team of health experts, we've put together the following list of best practices to keep your immune system primed for action and knock germs off their game. These tips are effective, easy to use, and even a bit unexpected. You needn't try all of them, of course—though the more you make part of your life, the better your chances of staying disease-free!

That's a Fact +

Your vacuum cleaner may not be as clean as you think. Because they suck up bacteria and food particles, vacuums can spread germs around your house. In a study at the University of Arizona, 13 percent of all vacuum cleaner brushes tested positive for *Escherichia coli*. To keep your vacuum cleaner clean, change the bag frequently—or, if you have a bagless model, clean the canister with bleach regularly.

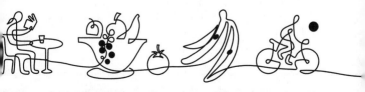

Eat Well, Stay Well

Just as your car needs gas and oil to run properly, your body depends on key nutrients to fuel its most basic processes, including your immune function. Your best strategy is to strive for the diversity of nutrients that comes only from a healthy, balanced diet, advises Ann G. Kulze, MD, founder and CEO of Just Wellness LLC and author of *Dr. Ann's 10-Step Diet*. Then, if you need to, add nutritional supplements to make up for any shortfall.

1 Eat for good health, not just immunity

Why it works A healthy diet nourishes your entire body, not just certain parts, explains David L. Katz, MD, MPH, director of the Yale Griffin Prevention Research Center in Derby, Connecticut, and author of *The Way to Eat*. "You need white blood cells for good immunity, and they require good bone marrow to form and a healthy heart and blood vessels to travel throughout your body," he says. "All of your body's systems are interrelated. That's why robust immunity equals robust health—and why healthy eating is really a holistic thing."

Where to start Your body will thrive on a diet that features whole grains, fruits and vegetables, and lean proteins such as chicken and fish. Nuts, seeds, olive oil, and avocados are good choices for monounsaturated fats. And don't forget fatty fish like salmon and mackerel for a healthy dose of omega-3 fatty acids.

What your body doesn't need are refined grains, sugars, and the saturated fats in red meats and full-fat dairy products. Try to limit these as much as possible.

For extra credit Here's a super-easy strategy to make sure that you're getting the proper mix of foods and nutrients at every meal. Imagine that your dinner plate is divided into quarters. Two of those quarters, or one-half of your plate, should be occupied by veggies and fruits. Then one-quarter is for whole grains, and the remaining one-quarter is for lean protein.

2 Pick brightly colored produce

Why it works Pretty much any fruit or veggie has something to offer your immune system. But for immune-boosting prowess, Dr. Kulze says, these are the cream of the crop: berries, whole citrus fruits, kiwi, apples, red grapes, kale, onions, spinach, sweet potatoes, and carrots. What do they have in common? Their eye-catching colors, which tell you at a glance that they're loaded with phytochemicals.

"The interesting thing about phytochemicals is that when they're isolated in supplement form, they seem to lose their immune-boosting benefits," Dr. Kulze notes. "That's why eating fruits and vegetables is the best strategy for getting the hundreds of micronutrients that work synergistically to enhance your immunity."

Where to start Choose fresh fruits and veggies when in season, frozen at other times of year. How you eat them is up to you! For example, you might sprinkle berries on your morning cereal, toss spinach and kale into a salad, or nibble on baby carrots for an afternoon snack. The possibilities are endless!

For extra credit Pair your produce with other healthy foods for a more powerful immune punch. You might mix your berries into yogurt containing active cultures, the beneficial bacteria that help keep the bad bugs in check. Or serve up a sweet potato as a side dish to wild salmon, which is rich in omega-3 fatty acids.

3 Be unconventional— go organic!

Why it works To most of us, a vegetable is a vegetable and a fruit a fruit. But some of our experts, including Neal Barnard, MD, president of the Physicians Committee for Responsible Medicine in Washington, D.C., believe that organic is the only choice if your goal is to ensure the robust function of your immune system.

One reason is that organic produce is more nutritious, with improved vitamin and mineral content, according to studies. Two, it contains fewer pesticides, among other chemicals.

Now the jury is out on just how harmful pesticides are. But in Dr. Barnard's opinion, "It's likely choosing organic products will result in lower cancer rates and, for women who are pregnant, fewer birth defects."

Where to start If you're still on the fence about organics, you needn't be a complete convert. Instead, try making the switch for just those fruits and veggies with the greatest pesticide content. As a general rule, peaches, apples, and bell peppers rank high for contaminants, while onions, avocados, and frozen sweet corn are largely contaminant-free. For a list of foods and their pesticide scores, visit www.foodnews.org.

For extra credit Before buying organic produce at the supermarket, check out what's available at your local farmer's market. "I am quite certain that I can find organic produce grown under large-scale farming conditions that is potentially less nutritious than produce grown locally," says Christopher Gardner, PhD, an associate professor in the Prevention Research Center at Stanford University School of Medicine.

4 Make omega-3s your favorite fat

Why it works Omega-3s help reduce inflammation, which is a factor in colds and flu, among many other conditions. If the latest research is any indication, that may be just one aspect of how these beneficial fats contribute to immunity. "Omega-3s are almost like the CEOs at the cellular level," Dr. Kulze says. "They create building blocks within the cells that drive the body's immune response."

Where to start Currently, there is no official guideline for omega-3 intake. To get the most from these beneficial fats, the American Heart Association recommends eating a serving of fish—particularly fatty fish like mackerel, lake trout, herring, sardines, albacore tuna, and salmon—at least twice a week.

For extra credit Although food should be your primary source of any nutrient, including omega-3s, Dr. Katz says this is one instance where supplementing may make good sense. "The typical American diet contains too many omega-6 fatty acids and not enough omega-3s," he notes. "A supplement can help restore proper balance."

Dr. Kulze likes a product called Nordic Naturals Omega-3D, which combines fish oil with another immune booster, vitamin D. To learn more about this product, visit www.nordicnaturals.com.

5 Use garlic liberally

Why it works Vampires aren't the only ones to be repelled by garlic. Bacteria and viruses are averse to its properties, too. The pungent bulb is an established germ fighter, and it enhances immunity besides.

Garlic owes its therapeutic properties to allicin, the chemical compound that's responsible for its very distinctive smell. Allicin increases both natural killer cells and T-lymphocytes, the white blood cells that seek out and destroy invading pathogens. "It's believed that people who ate a lot of raw garlic were the ones who survived the plague," says Susan Schenck, co-author of *The Live Food Factor*.

Where to start To get the most benefit from garlic, use the fresh stuff. "Fresh garlic that you mince yourself is a lot more potent than the dried or processed kind that you find at the supermarket," Dr. Kulze says. She recommends cutting it up about 10 to 15 minutes before you plan to use it.

For extra credit Eating raw garlic isn't for the faint-hearted; many people find the smell and taste overpowering. But cooking garlic can reduce its antimicrobial effects. If possible, try not to add it until the very end of the cooking process to help preserve its allicin content. Then stir it into soups and sauces, sprinkle it over fajitas and stir-fries, and use it as a garnish on steaks and burgers. Just remember, a little garlic goes a long way!

6 Add a little spice to your meals

Why it works The native cuisines of warmer, subtropical climates tend to feature a lot of spicy dishes, and for good reason. "The spices added to the food help keep it from spoiling, which prevents a lot of food-borne illness," Dr. Katz explains.

Many of these aromatic spices have potent antiviral properties. They're also excellent natural immune boosters, says nutritional consultant Steven Kushner, PhD. Because they work with your body's own immunity, they're less likely to cause the side effects that can accompany antiviral drugs.

Even the heat generated by certain spices has benefits. It clears mucus out of your nose and mouth while helping cilia work more efficiently, Dr. Kulze says. (Cilia are microscopic hairlike structures that line the respiratory tract and keep microbes from reaching your lungs.)

Where to start You can find hot and spicy dishes in many of the world's cuisines, especially Indian, Asian, and Mexican. Or simply experiment with various spices to find out how they might enhance the flavors of your favorite fare.

For extra credit Certain spices, such as cinnamon, cayenne, turmeric, and ginger, have been studied specifically for their antiviral properties, Dr. Kushner says. So find creative ways to incorporate these spices into your meals. Cinnamon gives a little kick even to plain old toast and applesauce, while cayenne is bold enough for barbecue and chili. Both turmeric and ginger are staples of Indian cooking—though for the less adventurous, a cup of ginger tea will do quite nicely.

7 Pay attention to vitamin D

Why it works Though much of the research on vitamin D is fairly new, all indications point to the nutrient being more important to our overall health than was previously realized. Among its growing list of benefits is its role in regulating immune function. An estimated 60 percent of Americans aren't getting enough vitamin D, and this may help explain why so many of us end up sick.

Where to start No doubt one of the reasons for our nationwide vitamin D shortage is its relative scarcity in our food supply. Fortified milk and breakfast cereals deliver the most generous amounts, as do fatty fish such as salmon, mackerel, and canned sardines and tuna.

The best natural source of vitamin D is the sun's ultraviolet rays, which your body converts to the nutrient. For this to work, though, you need to be out in the sun without sunscreen—and that's the rub for some experts, who are debating whether the benefits of brief sun exposure outweigh the risks.

For now, we recommend 10 to 15 minutes of unprotected sun exposure daily. If you're going to stay outdoors for longer than that, definitely slather on the sunscreen. Wear a hat and sunglasses, too.

For extra credit As for the omega-3s, you might want to consider taking vitamin D in supplement form, especially if you live in an area that doesn't get much sun. Many multivitamins provide the Daily Value (DV) of vitamin D, which is 400 IU.

8 Check your zinc intake

Why it works Zinc stimulates lymphocytes, a type of white blood cell that is critical to your body's natural defenses. It's one of the few nutrients that appears to play a direct role in shortening the duration of a cold.

Where to start For general immune enhancement, simply increase your intake of zinc-rich foods. Just six oysters provide five times the DV of the mineral, which is 15 milligrams. Other good food sources include lean protein (turkey and chicken), beans, and fortified cereals.

For extra credit If you think you may be coming down with a cold, start taking zinc at the first sign of symptoms. Studies suggest that zinc gluconate lozenges, such as Cold-Eeze, deliver more zinc into your body than other formulations, such as zinc citrate and thus are more effective.

9 Make the most of mushrooms

Why it works For more than 2,000 years, practitioners of traditional Chinese medicine have prescribed mushrooms to strengthen immune function. Now modern research is confirming the therapeutic properties of these versatile fungi.

For one recent study, conducted jointly by researchers at Pennsylvania State University and Arizona State University, five different kinds of mushrooms were incorporated into the diets of laboratory mice. When these animals were given a chemical that normally triggers colon inflammation and the growth of colon tumors, they showed no signs of adverse health effects. The reason: The mushrooms appeared to stimulate production of macrophages and T lymphocytes, two key cellular components of the human immune response.

Where to start These days, many supermarkets carry the various kinds of mushrooms traditionally used for medicinal purposes, including maitake, reishi, and shiitake. Interestingly, in the laboratory study mentioned above, the uncelebrated white button mushroom—the kind commonly used to top pizzas and salads—appeared to enhance immunity even better than the maitake or shiitake varieties.

For extra credit Fred Pescatore, MD, a traditionally trained physician who practices nutritional medicine and author of *The Hamptons Diet*, recommends a supplement called AHCC (short for active hexose correlated compounds). It's a blend of medicinal mushroom compounds that appears to have immune-boosting effects, according to studies conducted at Columbia, Harvard, Yale, and other institutions. Several formulations are available, but Dr. Pescatore prefers MushRex from Madre Labs and Kinoko Gold AHCC from Quality of Life Labs.

10 Give ginseng a try

Why it works Among herbalists, ginseng is what's known as an adaptogen, which means that it has broad-spectrum health effects. One species, North American ginseng, may be of particular benefit to the immune system. In a 2005 study involving 323 adults who had developed two or more colds in the previous year, taking North American ginseng supplement for 4 months reduced the number of colds, the severity of symptoms, and the number of days with symptoms.

The herb appears to get its immune-friendly effects from compounds known as polysaccharides. "These compounds stimulate macrophages and natural killer cells to release antimicrobial agents called cytokines," says Sherry Torkos, a pharmacist in Fort Erie, Ontario, and author of *The Canadian Encyclopedia of Natural Medicine*. "The cytokines directly attack viruses and bacteria and also activate immune cells that help protect the body against future attacks."

Where to start Ginseng is a popular ingredient in energy drinks, but these often contain large amounts of caffeine, not to mention other questionable substances. You're better off looking for a tea bag blend made with ginseng. Make the tea according to package instructions. Another option is to take 200 milligrams of a North American ginseng extract once or twice daily.

For extra credit A product called Cold-Fx has American ginseng as its active ingredient. It's available online and in many pharmacies.

11 Tap the power of probiotics

Why it works There might be something innately unappealing about intentionally consuming a food that contains (gulp!) live bacteria cultures.

Does it work?

Echinacea

Don't bother
For a 2005 study published in the *New England Journal of Medicine,* researchers gave 400 healthy volunteers either a placebo or one of three different doses of echinacea. After seven days of treatment, the volunteers were exposed to cold viruses via a nasal spray. Compared to the group given the placebo, the same number of people taking echinacea came down with colds. The dose didn't make a difference.

Echinacea is not without side effects, says Margaret Lewin, MD, clinical assistant professor of medicine at Cornell University and chief medical director of Cinergy Health. "It can cause drug interactions, allergic reactions, fertility problems, and abdominal pain and diarrhea," she says.

But these organisms are the good guys. They take up temporary residence in your gut, where they're able to counter the nasty effects of pathogens—the microbes that cause disease.

In a study of the probiotic *Lactobacillus reuteri*, only 11 percent of people given the probiotic took sick leave from work over the course of 80 days, compared to 26 percent of those given a placebo. The results were even more dramatic among people on night shift: No one in the probiotic group took sick leave, compared to 33 percent of the placebo group.

Where to start Dr. Kulze is a big fan of eating yogurt with live active cultures every day. It's an easy way to give your body the benefit of probiotics—and it's a source of protein and calcium that even people with lactose intolerance can stomach. "I recommend getting plain low-fat yogurt and mixing in your own fruit," Dr. Kulze says. "There's usually a lot of added sugar in the fruit varieties of yogurt." Look for the phrase "live active cultures" on the label.

For extra credit Scientific understanding of probiotics is becoming increasingly more sophisticated; doctors are now able to identify specific probiotics that are helpful for specific ailments. "Probiotics clearly have a benefit," Dr. Katz says. "This is a good example of when you should talk with your doctor—to find out what probiotic regimen might be right for you."

12 Stay hydrated

Why it works Like the rest of your body, your immune system depends on water to do its thing.

"When you're dehydrated, your immunity is compromised," Dr. Kulze says. "Your cilia don't function properly, your mucus doesn't do what it's supposed to, even your blood doesn't flow as well."

Where to start Let your body tell you how much water it needs. "The eight to ten 8-ounce glasses a day rule has been disproven," Dr. Katz says. "The more important guideline is to drink when you're thirsty. People who eat well tend to get plenty of fluids from fruits and vegetables, so they may not need as much water throughout the day."

Another good indicator of hydration is the color and frequency of your urine. "If you're getting enough fluids, you should urinate every 2 to 3 hours, and your urine should be a light straw color," Dr. Katz says.

For extra credit Don't forget to gargle! In a Japanese study involving 387 healthy volunteers, those who gargled plain water for 15 seconds three times a day reduced their chances of developing an upper respiratory infection by 36 percent compared to those who didn't gargle.

13 Drink two cups of tea daily

Why it works Tea is brimming with phytochemicals that seem to be the mechanism by which tea fends off illness. A recent study by Jack F. Bukowski, MD, PhD, looked specifically at ethylamine, a compound produced when the tea ingredient L-theanine is broken down in the liver. Dr. Bukowski found that when certain T cells were exposed to ethylamine, they multiplied 10-fold and were better able to fight off bacteria. Other research indicates that tea might play a role in battling viruses and parasites.

Where to start All tea seems to have immune-boosting properties, but research indicates that green tea trumps black—and white tea may be best of all. "Past studies have shown that green tea stimulates the immune system," says Milton Schiffenbauer, PhD, a microbiologist and professor in the department of biology of Pace University Dyson College of Arts and Sciences. "Our research shows that white tea extract can actually destroy the organisms that cause disease." Whichever variety you choose, Dr. Kulze recommends drinking at least two cups of freshly brewed tea a day.

For extra credit Drop a thumbnail-size chunk of ginger root into your tea—skin and all—and let it steep for an additional 3 to 5 minutes. Sip the tea with the ginger still in it, then chew on the ginger afterward. "Ginger goes great with tea and contributes even more anti-inflammatory and anti-viral compounds," Dr. Kulze says.

14 Practice safe food preparation

Why it works Though it makes headlines when our food supply is tainted in a factory or a restaurant, the reality is that most foodborne illness is caused by mistakes at home. Food gets left out too long; vegetables are contaminated by meat cut on the same surface; milk lingers in the fridge 10 days past its expiration date. Before you know it, you're hosting a breeding ground for bacteria and other nasty microbes.

Where to start The U.S. Department of Agriculture's Fight BAC! program distills the principles of safe food handling to four easy-to-remember guidelines: clean, separate, cook, and chill.

+ *Clean* your hands as well as any surfaces on which you'll be working before you begin preparing food.
+ *Separate* foods—especially raw meats—in the grocery cart, in the refrigerator, and when you're preparing a meal. This helps prevent cross-contamination.
+ *Cook* foods at the proper temperature and to proper doneness. You can use a food thermometer to check the internal temperature.
+ *Chill* foods at 40°F or below to prevent spoilage. Throw out any food that has sat out for more than 2 hours (or 1 hour when the air temperature is above 90°F).

For extra credit Visit www.befoodsafe.gov for more information about safe food handling, including proper cooking and chilling instructions for specific foods.

Move for Maximum Immunity

For weight loss and overall health, regular exercise tends to follow good nutrition on almost every expert's list. That's why in 2005, the USDA and the Department of Health and Human Services released their updated guidelines for physical activity. Thirty minutes a day used to be the standard, but now it's the bare minimum. Sixty to 90 minutes is the new goal.

Just as feeding your body properly gives it the

necessary fuel to fend off infection, moving your body regularly helps keep it resilient. "Exercise is a crucial component of immune function," affirms Erika Schwartz, MD, chief medical officer of www.healthandprevention.com. "During exercise, you release hormones called endorphins that stimulate your immune system. You also activate specific white blood cells that fight infection."

15 Exercise for 30 to 90 minutes every day

Why it works Moving your body affects your immune system directly and indirectly. For example, when you're under stress, your body releases stress hormones such as adrenaline, noradrenaline, and cortisol. They serve an important purpose, in terms of helping you to deal with stressors. But if they circulate in your system for too long, they can do more harm than good. When you exercise, you burn off stress hormones—which, in combination with those endorphins mentioned earlier, helps restore balance.

Where to start Any physical activity is good to start, especially if you've been relatively sedentary. Walking is a popular choice because it can be done virtually anytime and anywhere. Simple stretching, short bouts of bicycling, and yoga are other gentle activities to help ease you into a fitness routine.

For extra credit Although you definitely want to start slow, kicking up the intensity of your workouts is key to reaping their full benefit. "During exercise, your body temperature rises slightly, and this increase helps kill off bacteria and viruses," Dr. Schwartz explains. "Thirty minutes of aerobic or cardiovascular activity will achieve these effects. Slow walking and stretching will not."

16 Be careful not to overdo

Why it works Just as with red wine and dark chocolate, you can get too much of a good thing with exercise. "Research shows that more than 90 minutes of high-intensity endurance exercise can make people more susceptible to illness for several hours afterward," says Jenny Evans, a stress and fitness physiologist and founder of Power-House Performance Coaching.

This happens, at least in part, because of hormones. "Intense physical activity can trigger the release of stress hormones, which reduce long-term immunity," Evans explains. But excessive exercise has a much more basic impact on the body as well. "It can deplete glycogen and water and prevent the body from having the required energy for proper immune function," says Shane Ellison, MS, an organic chemist and author of *Over-the-Counter Natural Cures.*

Where to start Keep your workouts within the recommended 30- to 90-minute time frame. "Too much intense exercise can compromise immunity, but the average exerciser who does no more than 90 minutes per day has nothing to worry about," Evans says.

For extra credit If you do happen to fall ill after overexertion, the solution is easy enough: "Take time off to let your body repair and recharge itself," says Lou Schuler, a certified strength and conditioning specialist and author of six books, including *The New Rules of Lifting*. "Sometimes a cold or a bout of flu is a blessing in disguise, since it forces you to take a break from your workouts."

17 Do it for you

Why it works Exercise that improves your body shape also improves your self-esteem—and that's a good thing for your immune system. "The better you feel about how you look, the more confident you become, and the less stress you feel in various social circumstances," says Dr. Schwartz. "This leads directly to improved immune function, because stress lowers immune response."

Reality Check ✓+

The 5-second rule: When you drop a piece of food on the floor, if you pick it up within 5 seconds, it will still be germ-free.

Actually, 5 seconds is a bit on the conservative side, according to student researchers at Connecticut College in New London, who found that bacteria need more than 5 seconds to contaminate dropped food. For their study, the students left pieces of wet food (apple slices) and dry food (Skittles) on the floor for various periods of time, then analyzed the samples for contamination. It took 30 seconds for bacteria to find their way onto the apples; as for the Skittles, nearly 5 minutes elapsed before they were attacked.

Where to start The most effective workout for slimming down and shaping up combines aerobic activity with strength training. "Aerobic activity stimulates the release of endorphins, which increase your sense of well-being. But it's really strength training that builds muscle mass and improves your appearance," Dr. Schwartz says.

If you're new to strength training, it's a good idea to schedule at least a few sessions with a personal trainer, who can show you proper technique and tailor a workout to your skill level. And don't worry about becoming too muscular; you can get tone and definition without bodybuilder bulk.

For extra credit Focus on your core—that is, the muscle groups of your belly and your mid- and lower back. "Core strength training directly changes posture and thus enhances self-confidence," Dr. Schwartz says. She recommends abdominal exercises and Pilates classes to target your core muscles.

18 Sign up for a yoga class

Why it works "With yoga, it is not so much the activity itself but the destressing that goes along with it," says Walter Gaman, MD, managing partner of Executive Medicine of Texas and co-author of *Stay Young: Beating the Odds in a Busy World.* "Yoga is better for the body and mind because it incorporates both, unlike running on a treadmill, which works just the body."

In a small study at Washington State University, 19 breast cancer patients who took 8 weeks of Iyengar yoga classes showed reduced activation of

NF-kB, a protein that the body commonly activates when it's under stress.

Where to start Taking a yoga class from a certified instructor is the best way to get proper instruction in the movements and poses. If you don't have the time or finances to enroll in a class, the next best thing is a beginner's yoga DVD.

For extra credit To get a little variety and extra benefit, you can try different styles of yoga. The latest trend is something called Hot Yoga, in which you practice in a room heated to 95° to 100°F. "Hot Yoga can be challenging physically and thermally—a perfect combination for boosting immunity!" Ellison says.

19 Take your workout outside

Why it works Being outdoors can lift your mood, and a positive mood enhances the immune-boosting effects of exercise. "Exercising outdoors is fantastic," says Beth Shaw, a licensed yoga instructor and founder and president of YogaFit Training Systems. "If the air is fresh and clean, I will take an outdoor activity over an indoor activity any day of the week."

Dr. Gaman points out that when you're outdoors, you breathe in more fresh oxygen, which is fuel for your immune cells. And if the sun happens to be shining, those ultraviolet rays help your body manufacture another important immune booster, vitamin D.

Where to start It really doesn't matter what you do, though typically indoor activities like yoga and tai chi can be more effective when you take them outside. "Their healing benefits are magnified when they're performed by a body of water or in another natural setting," says Joseph Andreula, an owner of 18 gyms in New York and New Jersey and a member of the International Fitness Standards Advisory Council.

For extra credit Regardless of where you intend to exercise, check the air quality first. "Any form of activity will stress your immune system if pollution is high or ventilation is poor," Andreula says. "Ideally, you can exercise outdoors if the air is fresh and the climate is suitable, or indoors if the space is well ventilated."

20 Do what you love

Why it works Sticking with an exercise program is much easier when it involves an activity that you enjoy. "Any activity done regularly beats one that isn't done at all," Andreula says.

Where to start Think back to what got you moving as a kid. Was it riding a bike? Swimming? Dancing? Whatever it was, maybe you can pick up where you left off. Or perhaps there's an activity that you've been curious about. Now is as good a time as any to try it!

For extra credit Recruit a workout buddy or two. On those days when you're not feeling up to exercise, knowing that someone is counting on you can be motivation enough to keep your commitment. It's also an opportunity to strengthen social ties, a perk of exercise that gets little recognition for its immune-enhancing benefits.

21 Prep for exertion with vitamin C

Why it works Vitamin C has taken a bit of a beating since research revealed that it doesn't live up to its reputation as a potent cold and flu fighter. As often is the case, though, this "rule" has one exception: those who engage in strenuous activity. Across six studies involving 642 participants—including marathoners, skiers, and soldiers working in subarctic conditions—vitamin C supplements successfully reduced the chances of a cold by 50 percent.

Why this is true isn't quite clear, but Mark A. Moyad, MD, MPH, director of preventive and alternative medicine at the University of Michigan in Ann Arbor, has a theory. "When your body endures the oxidative stress that comes from a strenuous activity like running a marathon, it generates a ton of free radicals," he says. "So it makes sense that introducing a powerful antioxidant like vitamin C into the body would help to absorb some of that free radical damage and reduce its effects."

Where to start As mentioned earlier, your immune system can take a beating from long bouts of high-intensity exercise. So if you're expecting to engage in a strenuous activity—such as a charity 10K, or even a physically demanding job—you might want reinforce your natural defenses with a daily 400-milligram dose of vitamin C.

For extra credit Stick with the recommended dosage. While a little vitamin C may be good for your immune system, more isn't necessarily better. "Studies have shown that your body can't absorb more than 400 milligrams at a time," Dr. Kulze says.

22 Slim down if you need to

Why it works "Of all of the causes of depressed immunity, obesity is at the top of my list," Dr. Moyad says. "That's why I try not to discourage any form of activity. As long as people are doing something, they are taking steps toward getting healthier."

It goes back to Dr. Katz's idea of how one aspect of our health can influence all the others. People who weigh more than they should are more likely to be sedentary, to eat poorly, and to feel stressed—each of which contributes to depressed immunity. Studies confirm that reduced immune function is more common among those who are overweight or obese than among those who aren't.

Where to start To lose weight, you need to use more calories than you consume. So get moving, even if it's just a walk around the block at first. You have to start somewhere! What's important now is to focus on what you can do, not on what you can't, Dr. Moyad says. You'll be surprised by how quickly you see results, including on the scale.

For extra credit As your fitness level increases, continue to challenge yourself—whether by picking up your pace when you walk, or switching to heavier weights when you lift. You'll burn fat and build muscle, which together advance you toward your weight-loss goal—and give you a good immune boost besides.

Say Goodnight to Germs

Sleep just might be the Rodney Dangerfield of immune function: It gets no respect, at least as far as its contribution to restoring and sharpening our natural defenses. "Most people know what they must do as far as proper nutrition and exercise," says Carol Ash, DO, medical director of the Sleep for Life Center in Hillsborough, New Jersey. "They aren't so familiar with the basics of healthy sleep."

We need to take our sleep more seriously, because it's vital downtime that allows our bodies' various systems—including the immune system—to reboot. Even researchers have been surprised by just how big of an impact sleep has on immunity. "Our most important generator of energy is sleep," notes Barry Krakow, MD, a sleep specialist and author of *Sound Sleep, Sound Mind: 7 Keys to Sleeping through the Night*. "Sleep helps you to cope with stress, be productive, and avoid infection."

23 Make sure you get enough

Why it works In a nutshell, a certain amount of sleep is necessary to recharge your batteries each night. "Studies have demonstrated that getting

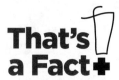

That's a Fact ✚

Freshly laundered clothes and linens may still harbor microbes. Disease-causing bacteria and viruses can linger even after clothes and linens have been washed and dried. To kill what's lurking in your laundry, wash underwear, bath towels, and kitchen linens separately, using hot water and chlorine bleach or a detergent that contains sanitizer.

less than an optimum amount impairs the function of immune cells that are important for fighting infection," Dr. Ash says.

The findings of a recent study involving 153 healthy men and women show how dramatic the effects of sleep can be, especially when it comes to fending off the common cold. After observing their volunteers' sleep habits for 2 weeks, researchers concluded that people who slept less than 7 hours a night were almost three times as likely to catch a cold as those who slept 8 hours or more.

Where to start As far as how much sleep you need, that's coded in your DNA, Dr. Ash says. While there is no universal number of hours that works for everyone, 7 to 9 is the usual range.{41}

"We do know that getting less than 7 hours is problematic for many of us," Dr. Ash adds. "A poll by the National Sleep Foundation found that 2 in 10 Americans get less than 6 hours of sleep a night"—a statistic that concerns most sleep specialists.

For extra credit You can prime your body and mind for a good night's sleep by allowing yourself an hour before bedtime to relax and reflect. Use this time to practice a few simple stretches or to meditate, which can help you unwind. You might want to consider investing in a white noise machine, which can help block out any background noise that can keep you from nodding off. These devices are widely available in retail stores and online.

24 Focus on quality, not quantity

Why it works Though many studies report on the number of hours of sleep because it's easy to track, Dr. Krakow agrees that the real issue is not how much you snooze but how well. When you don't get good-quality sleep, you're opening your body to all kinds of problems, including reduced immunity. "While you're sleeping, your body is oxygenating your blood and preparing you for another day," Dr. Krakow says. "When you don't sleep well, this oxygenation fluctuates, and your body hates that."

Where to start If you suspect that you might be a poor sleeper, ask yourself (or your bedmate) whether you snore, toss and turn, or wake up frequently—all classic signs of a bad night's sleep. Also pay attention to how you feel the next day. "You need to get a good assessment of your energy level," Dr. Krakow says. "Most people are so tired all the time that they don't even realize it. But if you step back and truly think about what your energy level is, you can get a sense of how tired you really are."

For extra credit It's not uncommon to have a restless or sleepless night on occasion. But if poor-quality sleep persists, schedule an appointment with your doctor or a sleep specialist. He or she can help pinpoint the problem and recommend a treatment plan to get you the truly good night's sleep that your body needs.

25 Clear up nasal congestion

Why it works The rattling and gurgling that's characteristic of clogged nasal passages can weaken immunity, and not just by disrupting sleep. "If you breathe poorly while you sleep, it wreaks havoc on your airways, causing irritation and inflammation in your nose and throat," Dr. Krakow says. "This leaves you more susceptible to colds and flu."

Where to start If you find yourself sneezing and sniffling during the day from allergies or other nasal irritants, taking care of this nose nuisance is a critical step toward sleeping soundly at night. Your doctor can recommend an appropriate regimen of allergy medication, nasal spray, and whatever else is necessary to ease your nighttime breathing. "You need to develop a zero-tolerance policy toward nasal congestion," Dr. Krakow says.

For extra credit Try Breathe Right nasal strips. "A lot of my patients have greatly improved their sleep just by wearing these strips at night," Dr. Krakow says.

26 Create an ideal sleep setting

Why it works Anything in your bedroom that doesn't directly pertain to sleep is a potential distraction. It can cause your mind to wander from the task at hand, which is to settle in for a long night of solid shut-eye. "Remove all possible stressors from the room that you sleep in," Dr. Schwartz advises. "Work stuff should never make it to the bedroom."

Where to start Start by clearing your bedroom of televisions, computers, and any other electronics. Reserve this space for sleep and sex—nothing else.

For extra credit Assess your bedroom decor; is it conducive to sound sleep? Dr. Ash recommends decorating with calming, soothing colors and comforting materials—including your mattress and pillows. Also, adjust your bedroom thermostat to a cool but comfortable temperature, anywhere from 54° to 74°F. The ideal temperature varies from one person to the next, but generally, a cool room helps to maintain sleep.

27 Make your room as dark as possible

Why it works The easy answer is that in a dark room, you're more likely to fall asleep and stay asleep. But Torkos says that the physiology is a little more complex than that. "In response to darkness, your body secretes a hormone called melatonin, which regulates your sleep cycle," Torkos explains. "Melatonin also supports immune function by acting as an antioxidant and by increasing the activity of T cells and the production of immune-stimulating interleukins and cytokines."

Where to start At the risk of stating the obvious, closing the bedroom door, pulling the shades, and turning out the lights all contribute to creating as dark a sleeping environment as possible. Turn an illuminated clock so that the dial faces away from you. If you can't completely darken your room— because of a nearby street light, for example—try wearing an eye shade to see if it helps.

For extra credit The benefits of sleeping in total darkness aren't worth hurting yourself by stumbling over something if you need to get up in the middle of the night. So keep a flashlight or low-wattage light at your bedside, just in case. "Unless you need a nightlight to maneuver without injury, it's best to learn to sleep without one," Dr. Ash says.

28 Obey your body's natural rhythms

Why it works Another reason to eliminate artificial night from your bedroom is that it allows your body to stick with its normal sleep-wake cycle. "Inside your brain is a clock of sorts that synchronizes your sleep-wake patterns," Dr. Ash says. "Light exposure at the same time every day sets this clock, called your circadian rhythm, to ensure consistent sleep and wake times."

Where to start Stick to a consistent sleep schedule, Dr. Ash advises. "After hours of wakefulness, a sleep-promoting substance builds up in your blood," she says. "When you maintain a consistent bedtime and wake-up time, the peak level of this substance correlates with the decline in the circadian rhythm for alertness, and you fall asleep. Interplay between these two processes also helps to wake you in the morning."

For extra credit Rise and shine—literally! Just as darkness is essential to set the "sleep" part of your sleep-wake cycle, light cues your body to ramp up for the day ahead. So don't stumble around in the dark after your alarm goes off. Open the shades to let in the sun; if you wake before sunrise, turn on your bedside lamp. Artificial light can do the job when natural light isn't available, Dr. Ash says.

Don't Worry, Be Healthy

Stress is an inescapable fact of 21st-century life. Whether our stressors are major (losing a job, ending a relationship) or minor (having a fender-bender, meeting a deadline), our bodies answer in the exact same way: Heart rate rises, breathing increases, digestion slows, among many other physiological changes. When stress is a constant, this so-called stress response never switches off. And that isn't good, especially for our bodies' defenses.

"The capabilities of the immune system are diminished with frequent activation of the autonomic nervous system, as is the case with chronic stress," says Jennifer Kelly, PhD, a licensed clinical psychologist at the Atlanta Center for Behavioral Medicine. "The immune system is downgraded so that it can continuously function."

29 Feel kneaded

Why it works Though research hasn't established a direct link between therapeutic massage and improved immunity, we can't think of a better antidote to stress than a little hands-on healing.

"When we are under stress, our bodies react by turning off the immune response," explains Barbara Stone, PhD, the author of *Invisible Roots: How Healing Past Life Trauma Can Liberate Your Present*. "Only when we're relaxed does the immune system have a chance to function properly. Massage is wonderful for this."

Where to start Think of a therapeutic massage not as a splurge but as an investment in your health. Be sure to find a professional with the proper credentials, whether it's state licensure or national certification (look for the initials NCTMB, which stands for Nationally Certified in Therapeutic Massage and Bodywork). Your doctor or local hospital may be able to recommend someone.

One caveat: You may not be a candidate for massage if you have an active infection, an injury, heart disease, cancer, or if you're at risk for blood

Does it work?

Face masks

Good bet (if worn by the person who's infected)
A face mask serves as a barrier to keep cold and flu viruses from spreading via saliva droplets. "So if you're sick and you sneeze, your droplets go into the mask and not into the air, which offers protection for the people around you," says Kathy J. Helzlsouer, M.D., M.H.S., director of the Prevention and Research Center at Mercy Medical Center in Baltimore.

A mask works best if it's worn by the person who's sick rather than by someone who's trying to avoid infection. Don't expect to be protected from other people's germs just because you're wearing a mask, Dr. Helzlsouer says.

clotting. Not sure if massage is right for you? Ask your doctor before beginning treatment.

For extra credit Dr. Stone recommends the following self-massage technique to relieve stress on the spot:

1. With your right hand, make a circle over your heart in a clockwise direction.

2. If you wish, add a counterclockwise circle on the opposite side of your chest.

3. As you do this, recite statements of self-acceptance, such as, "I deeply and profoundly accept myself with all my problems and limitations."

30 Learn how to relax

Why it works People who are under constant stress tend to have a hard time relaxing. Both progressive muscle relaxation (PMR) and biofeedback training can help defuse stress's effects—and boost immunity in the process.

PMR uses a combination of deep breathing and relaxation of the major muscle groups. "It's known that when you tense and relax your muscles, the effect is more profound than when you just relax," Dr. Kelly says.

In biofeedback, an external device evaluates various markers of stress—such as heart rate, skin temperature, and muscle tension—and conveys this information to you via visual or auditory cues. The idea is to use these cues to become aware of your physical state and consciously relax, effectively switching off your body's stress response.

Where to start PMR is easy to do on your own. As its name suggests, it involves tensing and then relaxing each muscle group in sequence, usually starting with your feet and moving up your body to your face. Until you get the hang of PMR technique, you might want to practice to an instructional CD. Many bookstores and libraries carry them.

For biofeedback, training with a licensed therapist is best. One common form of biofeedback involves an electromyograph, or EMG. If you're using computerized equipment, you'll see a line on-screen that represents muscle tension. Your job is to move that line, which you do by relaxing your muscles. That's how you learn relaxation.

For extra credit After you master these techniques, you can move on to others that require less time. One such technique is autogenic training, in which you release muscle tension with deep breathing. "The person creates a feeling of warmth and heaviness throughout the body and thus experiences a state of physical relaxation," Dr. Kelly says.

31 Make time for sex

Why it works When we make love, the brain releases a cascade of love-enhancing, stress-reducing chemicals, explains Frances Cohen Praver, PhD, an author and psychologist in private practice in Locust Valley, New York. Dopamine, for example, fuels our sense of pleasure, while oxytocin and vasopressin contribute to feelings of bonding and attachment.

A healthy sex life may influence immunity in a more direct way. Interesting evidence of this comes from a recent study at Wilkes University in Wilkes-Barre, Pennsylvania, for which researchers collected saliva samples from 112 students. Saliva contains immunoglobulin A (IgA), an antibody that helps protect against infection. The students also reported how often they were having sex. According to the researchers, those in the "frequent" group had the highest IgA levels of any group in the study.

Where to start In the Wilkes University study, "frequent" sex was defined as once or twice a week. That seems to be the optimum number for boosting IgA levels, at least compared to having sex less than once a week or abstaining.

For extra credit Don't overdo. Interestingly enough, IgA levels were lower among students who were having sex three or more times a week. As we've said before, you can get too much of a good thing.

32 Keep a journal

Why it works Think of a journal as your own personal therapist, without the bill. "Keeping a journal allows you to clarify your thoughts and feelings, thereby gaining valuable self-knowledge," Dr. Kelly says. "It's also a good problem-solving tool; you might hash out a problem and come up with a solution more easily when it's on paper."

Where to start Whether you use an ordinary spiral-bound notebook or a fancy leather-bound diary, what's most important is to get your thoughts and feelings on paper. Dr. Kelly recommends writing every day, while things are fresh in your memory. Some people like to carry their journals with them and take notes throughout the day.

For extra credit For keeping a journal to be beneficial, you need to write honestly and openly. Express your thoughts and feelings just as you would if you were in a private session with a therapist. "Journaling about traumatic events helps you to process them by fully exploring and releasing the emotions involved, and by engaging both hemispheres of the brain in the process," Dr. Kelly says. "This allows the experience to become fully integrated in your mind."

33 Whistle while you work

Why it works By one estimate, as many as two-thirds of us are unhappy with our jobs. That dissatisfaction can spill over into other aspects of our lives. "Constant preoccupation with job obligations often leads to poor eating habits and physical inactivity, resulting in weight problems, high blood pressure, and elevated cholesterol," Dr. Kelly says.

Yet considering that most of us spend roughly half of our waking hours at work, we need to find ways to make the best of a challenging situation. Otherwise, the stress can overwhelm our immune systems—and calling in sick just adds to the anxiety and tension.

Where to start No matter how unpleasant your work environment, you probably can find a colleague or two to commiserate with and lift your spirits. These relationships can help get you through the toughest times.

For extra credit See the humor in your situation. A study from Canisius College in Buffalo, New

York, confirms that humor helps people cope better with on-the-job stress. What's more, managers who use humor regularly are more effective and have more satisfied employees. If you're in doubt as to whether a joke is appropriate, always choose the safety of self-deprecation over poking fun at others.

34 Don't take job stress sitting down

Why it works "Jobs that require us to sit still all day, with very little opportunity to get up and move around, can hurt the immune system indirectly by impeding our ability to exercise," says Rallie McAllister, MD, MPH, co-founder and medical director of *The Mommy MD Guides* (www.mommymdguides.com) and a family physician in Lexington, Kentucky. To keep your job from lowering your resistance, fight back with stress-reducing, immune-boosting activities while you're at work.

Where to start Dr. McAllister recommends taking breaks as often as possible to do a few stretches, go for a short walk, jog up and down the stairs—whatever engages your muscles and short-circuits stress.

For extra credit If you do get sick, stay home! And take precautions to avoid picking up germs from under-the-weather co-workers, including washing your hands frequently and cleaning conference tables, keyboards, phones, and other shared surfaces with disinfectant. (For more strategies to avoid spreading infection in the workplace, see Chapter 3.)

35 Learn to say no

Why it works Women, especially, have a tendency to try to be everything to everyone—spouse, parent, friend, volunteer, the list goes on. In the process, we stretch ourselves too thin and leave too little time for ourselves. We can guess at the outcome: a cluttered, frustrated mind and a depleted immune system.

Where to start Saying no doesn't mean becoming a negative, nasty person. It's simply a matter of organizing, prioritizing, and very politely declining what doesn't fit into your schedule. "Become proficient at saying no to requests that aren't in line with your priorities," Dr. Kelly urges.

For extra credit People who have trouble saying no often don't realize how many obligations they have. So getting a handle on your commitments is an important step toward recognizing what you can and can't realistically do. "Staying organized and balanced will help you avoid overextending yourself," Dr. Kelly says. "This will reduce the amount of stress you experience and keep you healthier in the long run."

36 Flex your mental muscle

Why it works According to Dr. Kelly, stress doesn't just put a damper on immunity. It can muddle your mind, too, in the form of poor concentration, impaired short-term memory, and reduced productivity. Engaging and exercising your brain is a great way to fend off these negative effects from stress and enhance your immunity in the process.

Where to start Whether it's reading, doing crossword puzzles, or solving Sudoku problems, Dr. Praver recommends choosing an activity that you really enjoy. "Just make sure that it's something mentally active, not passive, like watching TV," she says.

For extra credit Try your hand at online brain games (we've posted a few of our favorites at www. prevention.com; click on Health, then on Brain Fitness). The one caveat with these: They shouldn't leave you feeling frustrated. If they do, they're just adding to your stress level, Dr. Rabin says.

Smile! It's Good for You

Remember the toy store slogan that promised shoppers to "turn that frown upside down"? You may want to take it to heart, for the sake of your immunity. According to a research review published in the September 2008 issue of the *Journal of Happiness Studies* (yes, there really is such a thing!), happy people are less likely to get sick than not-so-happy people. The effect of your mood on your physical health is more than skin-deep: It may increase the number and activity of key immune cells.

37 Maintain your social circle

Why it works As the song lyric goes, we all need somebody to lean on. Having a strong network of family and friends to share the good times and weather the bad can lift your mood—and your immunity. "Social support is as important for health and survival as low cholesterol and not smoking," says David Spiegel, MD, director of the Center on Stress and Health at Stanford University School of Medicine. "We are social creatures, and the absence of social contact is harmful to mental and physical health."

Where to start Dr. Kelly believes that you will be happier and healthier if you are constantly making an effort to expand your social network. "The more people you have in your life, the more likely you are to be in truly supportive relationships with at least some of them," she says. "It's beneficial to regularly add new people to your circle."

A good way to do this is to get involved in your community, says Bruce S. Rabin, MD, PhD, medical director of the Healthy Lifestyle Program at the University of Pittsburgh Medical Center. "What's important is not the number of friends you have in a single social context, but the number of social contexts in which you interact with people," Dr. Rabin notes. "Family, work, place of worship, book club, volunteer activities, sports activities—all provide opportunities for social interaction."

For extra credit Choose friends who reinforce your healthy habits. Surrounding yourself with people who support you is beneficial in its own right, but when you work together to be healthier, the effect is even greater. "Make a pact with them to encourage a positive attitude, good eating habits, and healthy choices," Dr. Gaman advises.

38 Turn on the tunes

Why it works Music puts you in a good mood, which in turn stimulates your autonomic nervous system (ANS) and kicks your immune system into gear. "The ANS can modulate virtually every aspect of immune function," Dr. Kelly says.

Where to start Tastes in music vary greatly from one person to the next. What matters most is that you listen to what you love. "Jazz, hip hop, classical, rock, country—it's your personal choice," Dr. Praver says.

For extra credit Composer Doc Childre recorded the album *Heart Zones* specifically to facilitate stress reduction and promote emotional balance. Research indicates that it just might work. In one study that compared the effects of 15 minutes of *Heart Zones* instrumental music against rock, New Age, and a period of silence, Childre's recording significantly improved immune function, especially levels of the antibody IgA. *Heart Zones* is available online and through music stores.

39 Watch a comedy

Why it works The simple act of laughing has multiple benefits for your immune system. It lifts your mood, reduces stress, and relaxes you, all of which keep your body's defenses sharp and primed for action. "Activities that produce deep belly laughter make the immune system more efficient at fighting off upper respiratory tract infections, activating T cells, increasing antibodies, and reducing stress hormones," Andreula says.

The therapeutic power of laughter has science in its corner. For one recent study, 33 healthy women were divided into two groups. One watched a funny video, while the other watched a tourism video. Across the board, the women in the humor group showed reduced stress and improved immune function, including an increase in natural killer cell activity.

Where to start Make time to laugh each day. Of course, laughter tends to be a spontaneous thing, but you can guarantee at least a few guffaws by watching a funny movie or TV show or listening to a CD by a favorite comedian. "Find things to do each day that are positive and fun," Dr. Gaman recommends.

For extra credit Yoga is good, and so is laughter, so why not put the two together? "Laughter Yoga is a program developed by a medical doctor in India, and it's wonderful," Dr. Stone says. To learn more, visit www.laughteryoga.org.

40 Discover your inner optimist

Why it works Some of us are "glass half-empty" people by nature. But with a bit of effort, it's possible to cultivate a more positive outlook. "You must consciously think of the good and not the bad," Dr. Gaman says. "When you catch yourself being negative, look for and verbalize something good about the situation. Over time, you can actually retrain your thought process."

Where to start Dr. Kelly offers this five-part technique to nurture a more positive mind-set:

+ Maximize your successes and minimize your failures.

+ Look honestly at your shortcomings, so you can work on them. Focusing on your strengths can also be helpful.

+ Keep in mind that the more you practice challenging your thought patterns, the more automatic it will become. It won't happen right away, but it will become ingrained over time.

+ Always remember that virtually any failure can be a learning experience and an important step toward your next success.

+ Give yourself a pep talk. You remember the story of *The Little Engine That Could*: He powered his way over a mountain that larger engines refused to climb, telling himself "I think I can, I think I can. . . ." Positive affirmations like this one can help you overcome obstacles, too.

For extra credit While it's healthy to look on the bright side at least on occasion, you shouldn't go to extremes trying to change who you are. That tends to backfire. "I've worked with a lot of CEO types who try to change themselves, and they end up miserable," Dr. Moyad says. "They may be driven to work long hours at the office, but that same personality is what makes them plan elaborate vacations and order flowers for their wives."

Create an Immune-Friendly Lifestyle

Our list would not be complete without the following strategies. Though they don't fit neatly into any one category, they can improve your chances of staying healthy not just during cold and flu season but all year long.

41 Know your family history

Why it works Your susceptibility to certain illnesses—from colds and flu to heart disease—may have a genetic component. But your genes don't necessarily have the final say in whether or not you get sick. By being proactive now, you may be able to reduce your risk in the long run.

Where to start Regardless of the ailments that may be tangled in your family tree, the fundamental advice remains the same: Take good care of your body generally, and your immune system specifically. By this point in the chapter, you know what to do!

For extra credit Target your self-care plan to the conditions that most concern you. "If you had a family history of heart disease, you would choose a diet of low-cholesterol foods to protect your heart," says Shawn M. Talbott, PhD, a nutritionist and author of *The Metabolic Method: The Complete Whole-Body Approach to Lasting Fat Loss, Better Mood, and More Energy*. "Likewise, if your family has a higher than normal incidence of colds and flu, then exercise, sleep, stress management, and selective supplementation may help reduce the frequency or severity of these illnesses."

42 Control your allergies

Why it works The sniffling, sneezing, coughing, and wheezing of seasonal allergies are bothersome in their own right. If mounting evidence bears out, allergies might undermine your health in other ways. "Allergies may predispose a person to infection," Dr. Gaman says. "This is probably due to an overtaxed immune system." So it makes sense that maintaining tight control of allergies could have a beneficial secondary effect of helping to keep colds and flu at bay.

Where to start To prevent the immune system drain that accompanies an allergy flare-up, the best approach is to avoid or manage your triggers. "Allergies are a form of inflammation, and inflammation is detrimental to the immune system," Dr. Praver says. "If you have allergies, research your offenders and stay away, or take an anti-allergy medication."

For extra credit Try quercetin. This powerful antioxidant, found primarily in the peel of apples and the outer layers of red onions, seems to have potent anti-allergy properties. "For folks with allergies, quercetin may be a viable alternative to some over-the-counter and prescription medications," Dr. McAllister says. "The compound has impressive antihistamine action, making it useful in the treatment of hay fever, eczema, and hives." To get your daily dose of quercetin, Dr. McAllister recommends heeding this timeless medical advice: Eat an apple a day—preferably a red one.

43 Get a flu shot

Why it works Most cases of seasonal flu could be prevented if everyone who's eligible for a vaccine actually got one. The vaccine works by

introducing a very small amount of the antici-
pated flu virus strains into your body. In response,
your body produces antibodies to those strains.
Then if by chance you are exposed to a flu virus,
your immune system is ready to respond.

As for rumors that getting a flu shot will give
you the flu, they're not true. Those who happen to
develop symptoms after getting vaccinated were
already infected with the flu virus.

Where to start The groups at greatest risk for
complications from flu—and therefore the leading
candidates for vaccination—are children, women
who are pregnant, people over age 50, those with
chronic health conditions, and residents of nurs-
ing homes. The vaccine isn't for everyone, however.
Among those who should avoid it are people with
allergy to chicken eggs; those with Guillain-Barré
syndrome, an autoimmune disorder; children
younger than 6 months; and anyone with an active
illness that involves fever.

For extra credit The vaccine against seasonal flu
does not prevent H1N1. For that, you will need a
separate shot. As of this writing, it is available only
to certain populations at high risk for infection.
Your best bet is to ask your doctor whether you're a
candidate. You can also get regular, reliable
updates on H1N1 and the vaccine supply by
checking the website for the Centers for Disease
Control and Prevention: www.cdc.gov/h1n1flu/.

44 Show your teeth some TLC

Why it works Think of your mouth as the "check
engine" light for the rest of your body. A problem

with your teeth or gums might be a sign of trouble elsewhere. The connection between the two isn't fully understood, but according to Howard E. Strassler, DMD, professor and director of operative dentistry at the University of Maryland Dental School in Baltimore, certain changes in the mouth can be an indicator of diabetes, kidney disease, stomach or intestinal problems, or a lung infection, among other conditions.

Where to start Practice good oral hygiene, including brushing your teeth at least twice a day (morning and night) and flossing at least once a day. "Another simple tip is to change your toothbrush if you have been sick," Dr. Gaman says. "This will keep you from reinfecting yourself." And be sure to see your dentist for a checkup every 6 months.

For extra credit Chronic bad breath is another potential signal that something is amiss in your body. "Bad breath due to a medical condition smells completely different than halitosis due to an oral condition," Dr. Strassler says. "If your breath ever has an unusual odor, you'll want to see your doctor."

45 Keep it clean— but not too clean

Why it works A warm, damp, dirty environment is like a "for rent" sign to germs. They won't feel quite so welcome if you regularly tidy up your living area and workspace. But don't overdo the fastidiousness, Dr. Spiegel says. "Exposure to pathogens boosts immunity," he explains. "There is some evidence that autoimmune diseases like asthma may be related to excessive cleanliness.

An immune system that isn't exposed to antigens may turn on its own body."

Where to start Certain surfaces should be cleaned and disinfected regularly to prevent infection. "The best way to avoid bad bacteria without the overuse of cleaners is to disinfect door handles, phones, and bathrooms at least once a week," Dr. Gaman says. "During flu season, you should be especially mindful of washing your hands after touching public objects such as door handles and shopping carts."

For extra credit While being neat can help reduce germ exposure, don't fret over messes. "Getting hung up on cleanliness will not benefit your immunity," Dr. Praver says. "If anything, the stress of always cleaning can reduce your immune function."

46 Winterize your immune system

Why it works There are reasons that seasonal flu is more prevalent in the winter months than at other times of year. For one thing, Dr. Rabin says, the flu virus grows best when body temperature is slightly below normal. That's more likely to occur as the outdoor temperature falls. For another thing, you're more likely to be indoors and in close contact with others, which makes spreading germs a whole lot easier.

Where to start As winter settles in, our healthy habits often go into hibernation. Exercise tends to suffer most—not surprisingly, since weather conditions can make outdoor workouts difficult. But staying active is extra-important at this time of year, as it strengthens immune function both directly and indirectly, by boosting your mood. "No matter how exhausted or depressed you are, exercise will make you feel better," Dr. McAlllister says. "Even a 20-minute walk, three times a week, can help keep you out of a serious slump."

For extra credit An even easier way to brighten your mood and head off an immune-depleting funk is to get some sun. "Just poking your head out the door or sitting in a sunbeam for a few minutes each day can help break up the winter doldrums," Dr. McAllister says.

If your winter blues are more persistent and unshakable, you may be dealing with full-blown seasonal affective disorder, a form of depression. In that case, you should see your doctor for proper diagnosis and treatment.

47 Turn down the volume

Why it works Excessive noise can have unexpected consequences for your immune system, mostly by raising your stress level. In European studies, traffic noise was shown to elevate levels of cortisol and other stress hormones, even during sleep. (Cortisol raises blood pressure and blood sugar while lowering immune response.)

Where to start If your work or home environment routinely exposes you to excessive noise, wear earplugs or headphones to help block it. Just be sure that doing so doesn't pose a safety risk.

For extra credit If the noise level is truly bad, you might want to consider a more extreme measure such as changing jobs or moving. "At least take regular breaks or small vacations from the noise," Dr. Gaman recommends.

48 Be wary of toxins

Why it works Environmental toxins challenge your immune system just as bacteria or a virus would. So when your body is putting all of its immune resources into undoing the effects of toxin exposure, it doesn't have much left to keep you from getting a cold or the flu. The most common sources of environmental toxins are household cleaners, impure drinking water, pesticide and insecticide residues on fruits and veggies, and mercury in fish.

Where to start You can reduce your toxin exposure by choosing "green" or natural household cleaners; getting your water quality tested periodically, especially if you have well water; and thoroughly washing produce before eating it (or buying organic). As for mercury, steer clear of king mackerel, shark, and swordfish, which have the highest mercury levels, according to the FDA. Anchovies, cod, clams, and crab have relatively low amounts.

For extra credit Drink lots of water to help flush away toxins and prevent their accumulation in the body's tissues. Give it a squeeze of lemon for a burst of antioxidants, which help enhance immune function.

49 If you smoke, quit

Why it works Cigarette smoke contains 43 known carcinogens. Knowing the damage that they can do to the rest of your body—heart disease, cancer, and emphysema chief among them—are you truly surprised that they wreak havoc on your immune system, too?

Once you quit, it's as though every cell of your being breathes a sigh of relief. Respiration, blood pressure, and blood levels of carbon monoxide improve within hours. Your risk of heart attack declines after one day.

Where to start You can improve your chances of quitting successfully by getting rid of all of your smoking paraphernalia—not just cigarettes but lighters and ashtrays, too. Tell everyone in your support network about your plans, so they can encourage you along the way. Try to steer clear of others who smoke, as well as situations that might tempt you to light up.

For extra credit Especially if you've tried to quit before, talk with your doctor about nicotine replacement therapy, in the form of patches, gums, lozenges, and sprays. It can help you get past the nicotine cravings and withdrawal symptoms that many smokers say are their main reasons for not quitting.

50 Use antibiotics responsibly

Why it works They certainly have lived up to their reputation as wonder drugs, but if antibiotics aren't used properly, they can open the door to more serious illness. That's because bacteria are able to adapt to their environments over time. If they mutate, they can become resistant to antibiotic treatment.

Consider tuberculosis as an example. This bacterial infection, usually of the lungs, is easily treatable with standard antibiotics. But those who contract an antibiotic-resistant strain of TB have a 40 to 60 percent chance of dying from the disease.

Where to start Antibiotics are effective only against bacterial infections. They should not be taken for anything else. (And if your doctor prescribes them to you for something other than a bacterial infection, don't be afraid to ask why.) If you are given a course of antibiotics, be sure to stay on it for the duration. Your infection may not be entirely gone even if your symptoms have subsided. Don't save or share antibiotics, and never use them as a preventive measure. They are meant only to treat an active infection.

For extra credit Go easy on antibacterial soaps and lotions. According to the FDA, these products are a major factor in the evolution of antibiotic-resistant bacterial strains. Wash up with plain old soap and hot water instead; it's just as effective at killing germs.

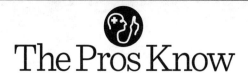

The Pros Know

Erika Schwartz, MD

Chief medical officer of www.healthandprevention.com

In her 30 years of practice, Dr. Schwartz has taken care of more than 100,000 patients, yet she rarely gets sick. Here's how she stays healthy:

First, I eat well—lots of fresh fruits and vegetables, no canned foods. I don't drink alcohol or soda—only water and green tea. I exercise every day and sleep 7 to 8 hours a night.

If I do feel like I'm getting sick, I take some extra steps to fend off whatever is trying to strike. For instance, I won't exercise that day, and I'll try to take it easy. Once I get home, I'll soak my feet in very hot water for 20 minutes. Then I put on a pair of socks and go to bed for 12 hours. Your immune system works much better when it has a way to drain viruses out of your system; putting your feet in hot water induces vasodilation and pulls things out. The Russian Olympic team does this when they are in competition and not feeling 100 percent. I also take about 800 milligrams of an immune booster called lactoferrin for five days.

When I was in my late twenties to mid-thirties, I didn't have to be as careful. My immune system was in great shape. But as I reached my late thirties and beyond, taking care of myself became even more important.

YOUR BACKUP PLAN

WHAT TO DO WHEN THE BUG BITES YOU

There's an old Italian saying that goes something like this: "Health is not valued until sickness comes." Indeed, when you're hunkered down in bed feeling too sick to move, probably the only thing on your mind is, how soon will you get better?

Hopefully, such occasions will be few and far between, now that you know what to do to take

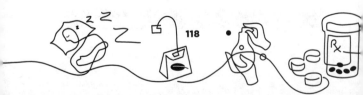

118

care of your immune system and minimize your exposure to germs. But if by chance a disease-causing bacterium or virus evades or overcomes your body's defenses, your priority will be to get back on your feet as soon as possible.

So consider this your "just in case" chapter—the one you hope you won't need, but you'll be glad to have handy if you do. We've asked our experts to share their favorite remedies for the most common microbe-borne illnesses, to help you recover quickly and reduce your chances of a repeat infection.

Colds & Flu

We so often mention colds and flu in the same breath that we may forget they're two distinct ill-nesses, with different viral causes.

The easiest way to tell whether you have a cold or flu is by the symptoms you're experiencing. In the case of a cold, they're largely respiratory—sore throat, coughing, sneezing, runny nose. Flu can have these symptoms, too, but it's much more likely to produce fever and chills, along with head-ache, muscle aches, and fatigue. "It comes on much more suddenly, and the symptoms tend to be much worse than with a cold," notes Christopher Czaja, MD, infection control officer for the National Jewish Health Hospital in Denver. Flu also can be more serious, especially for vulnerable populations like young children, the elderly, and those with chronic medical conditions.

Both cold and flu viruses spread from per-son to person via droplets from coughs and sneezes. These germs also like to hang out on

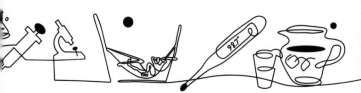

pens, telephones, computer keyboards—pretty much any surface that an infected person might touch. If you touch that surface yourself, then rub your eyes or scratch your nose, the virus is going along for the ride.

If there's any bright side to colds and flu, it's that they tend to clear up fairly quickly—in 3 to 10 days, in most cases. They do need to run their course, however, as medical science has yet to find a cure for either illness. These measures will help keep you comfortable in the meantime.

Lie down, fill up. "Get plenty of rest and drink lots of fluids," Dr. Czaja advises. "Drinking water helps thin mucous secretions in the lungs." What about that old standby, orange juice? It's fine as a fluid, but don't expect any bonus benefit from the vitamin C it contains. "I don't

RealityCheck ✓+

An apple a day keeps the doctor away.

In general, eating a healthful diet full of fresh fruits and vegetables is good for your immune system, says Kathy Helzlsouer, MD, MHS, director of the Prevention and Research Center at Mercy Medical Center in Baltimore. Apples, in particular, are rich in antioxidants and flavonoids; they also deliver an impressive 4 grams of dietary fiber each.

Research suggests that people who consume apples daily may be at lower risk for lung, colon, and breast cancer.

Still, when it comes to staying healthy, don't put all of your apples in one basket, so to speak. "By itself, an apple probably won't keep the doctor away," Dr. Helzlsouer says. "You need to eat and do other healthy things, too."

have anything against vitamin C, but the scientific studies have yet to prove that it's effective for preventing or treating respiratory infections," Dr. Czaja says.

Sip hot tea. All teas contain theophylline, which is a natural bronchodilator. So choose the brew that you find most tasty. Add a little honey, if you wish, says Gwen Huitt, MD, director of the Adult Infection Disease Unit at National Jewish Health Hospital. Honey contains antioxidants, which can help speed healing.

Reach for an OTC med. A pain reliever such as aspirin, acetaminophen, or ibuprofen can provide relief from fever and body aches, Dr. Czaja says. For a cough, look for a product that contains dextromethorphan. Guaifenesin is an expectorant that can help dislodge mucus. And pseudoephedrine is a very effective decongestant.

Get steam(ed). "Inhaling warm, moist air can help thin out and loosen mucus," Dr. Czaja says. You can make a mini steam bath by leaning your head over a bowl of hot water, being careful not to scald yourself. Or stand in a comfortably hot shower.

Cover your mouth. "Cough into a tissue, then toss it," Dr. Czaja suggests. "If you don't have a tissue, cough into your sleeve, then wash your hands." If you're bringing up thick, green mucus, you probably have a bacterial infection in your airways, in addition to the respiratory virus. This calls for a trip to the doctor; he or she may prescribe antibiotics to clear up the infection.

Choose your company carefully. Once you're feeling better, you can greatly reduce your chances of reinfection by avoiding close contact with anyone who has a cold or the flu. If that just isn't possible, then the next best thing is to wash your hands constantly and thoroughly, or use an alcohol-based hand sanitizer if you're not close to a sink.

Schedule a vaccine. The best way to stop the flu from spreading to you is to get vaccinated. Because flu strains vary from year to year, you need the vaccine annually. It's administered as an injection or a nasal spray. Though it may be available as early as September, you can get vaccinated any time during flu season, which may continue through early spring.

Ask your doctor about a flutter valve. If you're prone to respiratory problems or you tend to produce a lot of phlegm, you might be a candidate for a device called a flutter valve. It helps loosen mucus so that it's easier to cough up. Your doctor can tell you more about it.

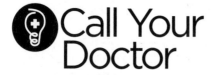

Call Your Doctor

Any of the following signs and symptoms requires medical attention:

✚ Fever above 101.5°F

✚ Shaking chills

✚ A cough with phlegm that doesn't improve or worsens

✚ Bloody sputum

✚ Shortness of breath with normal daily activities

✚ Chest pain when you breathe or cough

✚ Unable to keep down food or liquids

Food Poisoning

You might know *Attack of the Killer Tomatoes!* as a campy horror flick. But the title could just as well apply to any of the 76 million cases of food-borne illness that occur in the United States each year, according to the Centers for Disease Control and Prevention. They're the end result of consuming foods or beverages tainted with pathogenic organisms—usually bacteria such as *Escherichia coli*, salmonella, and shigella, but sometimes viruses and parasites.

Raw, ready-to-eat foods such as lettuce greens, spinach, radishes, and yes, tomatoes are the most common sources of food poisoning, says Amy Foxx-Orenstein, DO, a gastroenterologist at the Mayo Clinic, and immediate past president of the American College of Gastroenterology. "They may grow in fields where pasture animals walk and graze, and their water becomes contaminated with animal feces," Dr. Foxx-Orenstein explains. Raw meat and poultry can become contaminated during processing, packing, and shipping. Some foods pick up pathogens when they're prepared on unclean surfaces or allowed to sit out too long.

If you have the misfortune of consuming one of these foods gone bad, you'll know by the unmistakable symptoms: upset stomach, diarrhea, abdominal cramps, vomiting, fever, and dehydration. While onset may be within a few hours, that isn't always the case. "Some cases of *E. coli* have been traced back a week," Dr. Foxx-Orenstein says. "With other contaminants, you may need to go back a month."

The symptoms are miserable, to be sure, but your body is doing what's necessary to get rid of the offending organism. Here's how you can help it along.

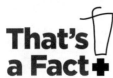

That's a Fact

Replenish fluids. "The most serious complication from food poisoning is dehydration," Dr. Foxx-Orenstein says. "All that diarrhea and vomiting causes you to lose fluids, electrolytes, minerals, and essential salts." She suggests sucking on ice chips or sipping water, a sports drink, or diluted fruit juice. Ginger ale and hot ginger tea are other good choices; just be sure that the soda has gone flat. "Carbonation creates bubbles in the stomach, which contributes to gastrointestinal distress," Dr. Foxx-Orenstein explains.

Move on to bland foods. Once you feel up to it, try the so-called BRAT diet, which consists of bananas, rice, applesauce, and toast—all gentle on the gastrointestinal tract. Gelatin, crackers, and toast also go down easy. If you feel at all nauseous when you eat, switch back to your liquid diet for a bit longer. Your digestive system may not be up to solid foods just yet.

Hold off on the meds. As much as you might want to, don't take an anti-diarrheal, at least not right away, Dr. Foxx-Orenstein advises. You want your body to flush out the offending organism, but an anti-diarrheal will inhibit that process, allowing the toxin to linger even longer. "If you're still having diarrhea after 48 hours, then try an OTC product," Dr. Foxx-Orenstein says.

Handle food with care. Once you've been

through one bout of food poisoning, you'll likely do whatever is necessary to prevent another. The easiest and smartest strategy is to make sure that everything you eat (and drink) is properly prepared and stored. Specifically:

✚ Wash your hands frequently when you're handling food.

✚ Keep raw meats, poultry, and seafood separate from ready-to-eat foods to avoid cross-contamination.

✚ Don't use a wooden cutting board. Grooves in the wood can harbor bacteria.

✚ Cook food to an internal temperature of 165°F to kill off any microbial growth. You can check the temp with a cooking thermometer.

✚ Refrigerate uneaten food immediately. If it's left to stand at room temperature for more than 2 hours, it may not be safe to eat.

✚ Set your refrigerator temperature at 40°F or lower, and your freezer at 0°F.

For more tips on safe food handling, see Chapter 3.

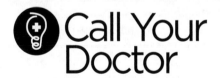

Call Your Doctor

See your doctor promptly if food poisoning is accompanied by:

✚ Fever above 101.5°F

✚ Blood in the stool

✚ Diarrhea that lasts more than 3 days

✚ Prolonged vomiting that prevents you from keeping down even liquids

Gastroenteritis

Even though it's the second most common infectious illness in the United States, according to the National Institutes of Health, gastroenteritis has long suffered an identity crisis. For one thing, it's often called the stomach flu, even though it has no connection to the influenza virus. The most common causes are bacteria such as *Helicobacter pylori*, salmonella, shigella, and giardia, as well as viruses such as norovirus, which was responsible for the recent spate of outbreaks on cruise ships.

On top of that, gastroenteritis is frequently mistaken for food poisoning because of its most prevalent symptoms: diarrhea, vomiting, abdominal pain, and fever. It usually runs its course in a day or two, although for an unfortunate few, symptoms can linger for up to 10 days.

Just as with food poisoning, your body needs to eliminate whatever is causing your gastroenteritis. This means staying close to the bathroom, at least until your symptoms start to let up. The main goal of treatment is to replenish lost fluids and nutrients.

Sip, then sip some more. Pretty much any beverage will do, as long as it isn't caffeinated. Caffeine can irritate the stomach lining, which is what you don't want right now. Water, sports drinks, fruit juice, ginger ale, and decaf tea are all good choices, Dr. Foxx-Orenstein says. As for how much to sip, it depends on how severe the infection is and how much you can tolerate. Start slowly and increase your intake very gradually.

Switch to solid foods when you're ready. You don't want to rush this step; if you try to eat too much too soon, whatever goes down may come back up pretty quickly. As for food poisoning, our experts recommend starting out with the BRAT diet, which consists of bananas, rice, applesauce, and tea—all bland, easily digestible foods.

By all means, keep your hands clean. Gastroenteritis is highly contagious, and it's usually spread by people not washing their hands, Dr. Foxx-Orenstein says. You can do your part to avoid passing on the infection to someone else—and to protect yourself from a recurrence—by washing your hands often, especially when you're in contact with public surfaces such as door and shopping cart handles. Keep an alcohol-based hand sanitizer with you for those occasions when you may not have ready access to soap and water.

Traveling? See your doctor for a vaccine. So-called traveler's diarrhea is a form of gastroenteritis. Especially if you're heading to a locale with questionable sanitary practices, it's a good idea to get vaccinated against gastroenteritis carriers like salmonella, typhus, cholera, and rotavirus.

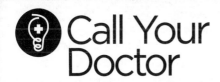

Call Your Doctor

With garden-variety gastroenteritis, you should start feeling better in a day or two. See your doctor if you experience any of the following:

✚ Symptoms last for more than 3 days

✚ Dizziness upon standing

✚ Blood in vomit or stool

✚ Fever above 101.5°F

✚ A swollen abdomen or abdominal pain emanating from the lower right side

✚ Little to no urination, extreme thirst, and dry mouth

Sinusitis

At first you think you're dealing with a classic case of the common cold. But then 10 days or so pass, and you're not feeling any better. If anything, your symptoms—nasal congestion and postnasal drip, sore throat, cough, fever, facial pressure—seem to be settling in for the long haul. That's what often happens with a sinus infection, or sinusitis. (The suffix -*itis* means inflammation.)

Most cases of sinusitis are the result of a viral infection, says Andrew Lane, MD, director of the Division of Rhinology and Sinus Surgery at Johns Hopkins School of Medicine in Baltimore. Though sometimes the viruses are airborne, usually they're transmitted by hand-to-hand (or hand-to-contaminated-object) contact. Less than 1 percent of sinusitis is caused by bacterial infection, Dr. Lane says. That's a good thing, because when it happens, bacterial sinusitis can last 4 weeks or longer. Viral sinusitis usually clears in about 10 days.

Whatever the cause of your sinus infection, these tips can have you breathing easier in no time.

Turn up the humidifier. "The nose is very sensitive to humidity in the air," Dr. Lane says. "When moisture is low, it contributes to nasal congestion. A humidifier warms and moistens the air, so it's easier for the lungs to handle. This will help reduce congestion, too."

By the way, Dr. Lane says not to bother putting mentholated products in a humidifier or in hot water to help open nasal passages. "Studies have shown that this practice doesn't really increase lung capacity," he notes. "It just creates a tingly sensation in your nose, which gives you the impression that air is moving through your passages faster."

Choose OTC meds carefully. These days, drugstores have entire aisles of products that promise to open clogged sinuses and relieve congestion. They can help, but only if you pick the right product for your symptoms. If you're dealing with nasal congestion, for example, you'll want to look for a product that contains oxymetazoline, a decongestant.

"Some people mistakenly buy cold medicines that contain antihistamines," Dr. Lane says. "Antihistamines can thicken mucus, dry out the sinuses, and make you sleepy. They're helpful for allergies, but not for a sinus infection."

Rinse out your sinuses. If you'd prefer a nonchemical remedy to your sinus infection, ask your pharmacist to suggest an OTC preparation

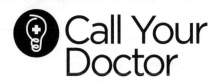

Call Your Doctor

Viral sinusitis tends to run its course in about 10 days. If your symptoms persist longer than that, you may be dealing with a bacterial sinus infection. You should see your doctor for proper diagnosis and treatment, which likely will include antibiotics. Also see your doctor if you have:

✚ Fever above 100°F

✚ Multiple episodes of sinusitis in a year's time

✚ Symptoms that do not respond to treatment with OTC products

✚ Vision changes

✚ Lethargy

that's essentially a saline nasal spray. "You can also use contact lens solution," Dr. Lane says. "Sprayed into your nose, it helps flush away irritants, along with any thick mucus that's sitting there causing trouble."

Increase your fluid intake. Being dehydrated only aggravates nasal congestion. "Dry mucus membranes don't allow your sinuses to move the mucus efficiently and clear the infection," Dr. Lane says. He recommends drinking between 8 and 10 glasses of fluids a day for the duration of your sinusitis.

Relax. "I know it isn't easy to slow down, but if you continue to function at the same level while you're sick, you won't recover as quickly," Dr. Lane says. "You need to give yourself a little time and take care of yourself."

Strep Throat

Strep throat is no ordinary sore throat. Caused by group A streptococcus bacteria, strep tends to come on quickly and painfully. The simple acts of talking and swallowing suddenly are not so simple. "If you could see into your throat, it would be red, with white patches on your tonsils," Dr. Lane says. "You also might have swollen lymph nodes and/or neck tenderness, fever, headache, and fatigue."

Anyone can get strep throat, but it's much more common in kids between ages 5 and 15. A crowded environment, like a daycare or a school, is ideal for spreading the bacteria from one person to another.

If you suspect that you have strep throat—especially if sore throat symptoms last 3 days or longer and seem to be getting worse over time—you should schedule an appointment with your doctor. He or she will swab your throat to confirm that it's strep; if it is, you'll likely be given a course of antibiotics to help clear the infection. Try these strategies for additional relief.

Pamper your throat. "Getting plenty of fluids will moisten soft tissue in the throat, which can help alleviate pain," Dr. Lane says. "My patients tell me that warm fluids seem to be more soothing."

Be very, very quiet. You probably won't feel much like talking anyway, but your throat needs to rest. So try to use it as little as possible while you're on the mend.

Cruise the cold-care aisle at the drugstore. OTC pain relievers such as aspirin, acetaminophen, and ibuprofen can relieve the pain and fever that accompany sore throat. Lozenges and throat sprays are also effective.

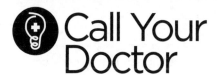 # Call Your Doctor

See your doctor promptly if you experience:

✚ A painful sore throat that lasts 3 days or longer

✚ Hoarseness that lasts longer than 2 weeks

✚ Difficulty swallowing or breathing

✚ Fever above 100°F

✚ A rash along with your sore throat

✚ Blood in your saliva or phlegm

✚ Symptoms of dehydration (i.e., dry mouth, reduced urination, dizziness, or lightheadedness)

✚ Recurring sore throats

Take all of your antibiotics. You need to finish your entire prescription, even if you start to feel better. Otherwise, the infection can recur and the complications can be severe, Dr. Lane says.

Urinary Tract Infection

When you gotta go, you gotta go—and with a urinary tract infection (UTI), the urge is almost constant. Even worse is the intense pain and burning on urination, which might make you put off going for as long as possible. You may notice blood or cloudiness in your urine, too.

A UTI occurs when wayward bacteria—often *E. coli*—find their way into the urinary tract, where they grow and multiply. Thanks mostly to anatomical differences in the genitourinary tract, women are way more likely than men to get UTIs. In fact, according to the National Kidney Foundation, one in every five women develops at least one UTI in her lifetime.

With antibiotic treatment, most UTIs clear up within a day or two. You can keep your recovery on track, and future UTIs at bay, by heeding this advice.

Drink lots of water. This will help flush out the harmful bacteria. An easy way to know if you're getting enough water is to check the color of your urine; it should be a very pale yellow, says Linda Brubaker, MD, director of the urogynecology division for Loyola University Health System.

If you drink a lot of coffee, you'll need even more water, because the caffeine in coffee acts as a diuretic. Also increase your water intake if you're very active or you live where it's hot and dry.

Add cranberry juice to your self-care regimen. Although cranberry juice hasn't lived up to its reputation as a UTI fighter, it appears to be effective as a preventive. When University of Minnesota researchers reviewed data from several studies, they determined that cranberry juice can reduce UTI recurrence by about 35 percent in young and middle-age women.

According to Jill Maura Rabin, MD, head of the urogynecology department at the Long Island Jewish Medical Center in New Hyde Park, New York, and author of *Mind Over Bladder*, cranberry juice acts as a detergent of sorts, helping to maintain a low pH in the urinary tract. This creates an unfavorable environment for bacteria. Her advice: If you're in the category of women who's prone to UTIs, drinking cranberry juice certainly can't hurt, and it just might help.

Practice good hygiene. It's a good idea to change sanitary pads and tampons frequently, Dr. Rabin says. "Because the vagina and bladder sit side by side, heavily saturated pads and tampons can encourage harmful bacteria to travel up into the urethra," she explains.

Consider an estrogen cream. For women at or past menopause, declining estrogen levels can

That's a Fact

Teachers have the germiest profession. University of Arizona researchers found that the phones, keyboards, and desks used regularly by teachers, accountants, and bankers housed 2 to 20 times more bacteria per square inch than the same equipment used by other professionals. Teachers' phones were the worst source of bacteria, followed by their desks, keyboards, and computer mice. Accountants' and bankers' equipment ranked second and third, respectively.

raise the risk of UTIs by causing pelvic tissue to thin and dry out, leaving it more susceptible to harmful bacteria. "Some women who get a lot of UTIs benefit from using an external estrogen cream," Dr. Brubaker says. "The estrogen thickens the walls of the urinary tract and vagina, so bad bacteria don't get a foothold as easily." Ask your doctor whether an estrogen cream might be helpful for you.

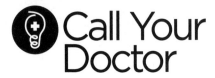

Call Your Doctor

If you repeatedly get what seem to be symptoms of a urinary tract infection (UTI), you should see your doctor. You may have another pelvic condition that requires a different course of treatment. Other symptoms that require a doctor's attention if they occur with a UTI include:

✚ Blood in your urine

✚ Fever and chills

✚ Lower back pain

✚ Nausea and vomiting

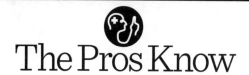

The Pros Know

Ken Munson

Sanitation and infection control specialist for the
Munson Group and specialized consultant to
BioTech Medical, North Canton, Ohio

Since his job requires him to spend a lot of time in hospitals, schools, and other public facilities, Munson is diligent about following personal hygiene protocols, especially during flu season.

First, I get the flu vaccine as soon as it becomes available. I eat as healthfully as I can, and I stay active by playing tennis three times a week and working out at the gym as often as it fits into my schedule. I make a conscious effort to limit the number of times I touch my face, nose, mouth, and eyes to reduce the chances of transmission.

I frequently wash my hands in warm water for at least 15 to 20 seconds, making sure to produce a good lather. When I can't wash my hands, I use an antimicrobial sanitizer. The antibacterial products don't kill the viruses that cause flu and some gastrointestinal illnesses.

When I'm on the road and staying in a hotel, the first thing I do is disinfect the TV remote as well as the bathroom faucets and the toilet flush handle with my own bottle of SpectraSan 24. I try not to touch elevator or vending machine buttons with my fingers; I use my knuckle or elbow instead. Hundreds of people press these buttons, which are rarely cleaned and disinfected. I also try to avoid holding onto escalator rails.

I'm not a health nut, but I do what's practical. These measures don't guarantee that I won't get sick, but they certainly reduce my chances.

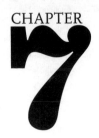
THE KIDS AREN'T ALRIGHT

*SAFEGUARDING YOUR FAMILY
AGAINST INFECTION*

If kids came with any sort of instruction manual, it would need an entire section devoted to the various infectious ailments that they're likely to bring home. The fact is, kids are magnets for germs. The littlest ones put their hands—and mouths—on just about anything. Older ones aren't quite so

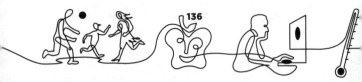

indiscriminate, although they still can be rather haphazard with their personal hygiene. They might cringe at a kiss from Mom or a hug from Dad, but they won't hesitate to share water bottles, lip balms, and toothbrushes with their BFFs.

Not to mention that kids spend most of their waking hours in places teeming with germs. A survey of schools by the public health and safety organization NSF International found water fountain handles and spigots, computer keyboards, and even basketballs to be crawling with bacteria.

It's no wonder, then, that your offspring might seem to be under the weather more often than not. The average school-age child comes down with five or six colds a year, while younger kids gets as many as eight. Infants are especially vulnerable to infection; the reason is that by the time they're about 8 months old, they're exhausting the antibodies that they received from their moms while in the womb and breast-feeding, and their own immune systems are still ramping up.

When Your Child Gets Sick

As hard as you may try, you likely won't be able to protect your child from every bug that comes down the pike. Thankfully, the infectious illnesses most common among the younger set tend to be relatively mild and go away on their own. To keep kids comfortable and their germs confined, heed this expert advice.

Resist the urge to rush to the doctor. It frustrates parents, but doctors don't want them to

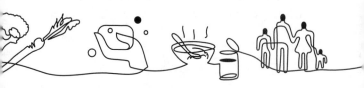

bring their children into the office for every cough and sniffle, says Mary Elizabeth Romano, MD, a pediatrician and assistant professor of pediatrics at the Monroe Carell Jr. Children's Hospital in Nashville. Why? Because ordinary colds and flus need to run their course and can't be cured with antibiotics. Besides, just sitting in the waiting room with all those other patients exposes kids to germs that could make them even sicker.

Keep them home while they're contagious. During cold season, runny noses can be as common as backpacks in schools. But certain signs and symptoms may warrant a sick day. Laura Jana, MD, a pediatrician in Omaha, Nebraska, and a member of the executive committee for early education and childcare for the American Academy of Pediatrics, recommends a day at home if your child:

- ✚ Is vomiting or has diarrhea
- ✚ Has had a fever of higher than 100°F in the past 24 hours
- ✚ Is showing signs of more than a common cold, such as a bad cough

Keep in mind, too, that when kids are too sick to go to school, then they're also too sick to go to a friend's house or out for dinner, Dr. Romano says.

Let them know it's not time for sharing. When your child is sick, discourage him or her from sharing cups, utensils, towels, and toothbrushes with siblings, Dr. Romano advises. Baths and sleeping arrangements should be separate, too.

Fill their tummies with chicken soup. Science has shown that chicken soup really does help fight a cold by reducing the inflammation that occurs with a viral infection. Can't get your child to eat it? Try putting the broth in a cup with a straw.

Corralling What the Kids Dragged In

Once your child is feeling better, you may think you're home free. Not so fast! Just like grownups, kids can carry and spread germs even when they're symptom-free. And while your child may be able to withstand certain pathogens, others in your household may not be so lucky.

The simplest, cheapest solution to keep illness from becoming a family affair is regular, thorough

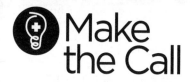

Make the Call

While it's true that not every childhood infectious illness requires a doctor's visit, the following should be your cue to pick up the phone and schedule an appointment:

✚ Any fever in an infant 6 months or younger

✚ Rapid or distressed breathing

✚ Extreme fatigue or difficulty waking

✚ Vomiting and not tolerating food

✚ Acting out of character

✚ A cold that lasts longer than 7 to 10 days and seems to get worse rather than better

If you aren't sure what to do, call your doctor's office and ask to speak with a nurse about your child's symptoms.

hand-washing. Teach kids to scrub up as soon as they enter the house, before and after eating, after using the bathroom, after coughing or sneezing, after playing with pets, and after being around someone who's sick. They will notice if you aren't practicing what you preach, so be sure to set a

The Antibiotic-Asthma Link

Nearly 5 million American kids have asthma, and if current predictions hold true, that number could mushroom to 100 million by 2025. What's behind the explosion in asthma cases? Some research is pointing a finger at the rise in antibiotic use.

In a 2007 study involving more than 13,000 children in Manitoba, Canada, those kids who took more than four courses of antibiotics during their first year of life were 1½ times as likely as other kids to develop asthma. Another study, this one involving 448 children, found similar results when kids were given at least one course of antibiotics before their 6-month birthdays.

Some experts suspect that antibiotic treatment could alter how a child's immune system develops, increasing asthma risk. Others aren't so sure—and some studies failed to find an antibiotic-asthma link.

The best advice for concerned parents is to practice prudence in their antibiotic use, counsels Vivian Lennon, MD, medical director of primary care for Children's Healthcare of Atlanta. That means giving antibiotics to kids only for infections known to be caused by bacteria, fungus, or parasites, such as ear infections or strep throat. Antibiotics are not effective against viral infections such as colds and flu.

good example. (For a refresher on good hand-washing technique, see page 28.)

Here are more strategies to keep germs contained and your whole family healthy.

Roll up the welcome mat. Designate a spot near the door where kids can leave their backpacks and shoes when they get home from school. Then you can clean the backpacks with a disinfecting wipe or spray before they get dragged through the rest of the house.

Wipe down daily. Dr. Jana suggests sanitizing those surfaces where your kids are most likely to come into contact with germs: the kitchen counter and table, the kitchen and bathroom sinks, the toilet (including the handle), and doorknobs and light switches. A daily once-over with disinfecting spray or wipes is all that's needed, except for surfaces on which you prepare food; those should be sanitized before and after each use.

Teach them proper cold etiquette. The droplets produced by a sneeze or cough can travel through the air and land in someone else's mouth or nose. It's how cold and flu viruses usually spread, experts say. To keep germs from going airborne, train your kids to sneeze into tissues and cough into their elbows.

Keep little hands out of little mouths. This may be easier said than done, as toddlers will suck, bite, and chew on just about anything. But every time they do, they're getting a mouthful of germs, too.

Sneaky Ways to Shore Up Immunity

There's one more way to protect your child (and the rest of your family) from the current crop of germs, and that's to strengthen his or her natural

That's a Fact

Want ketchup with your fries? You may be getting a dollop of bacteria, too. In a typical busy restaurant, more than 40 people may touch a single ketchup bottle on any one day. The condiment containers seldom get wiped down with the rest of the table. So if you reach for a french fry after handling the ketchup, you could be picking up whatever germs were left behind by the diners before you. To reduce your risk, clean your hands with an alcohol-based sanitizer after handling any condiment container, including salt and pepper shakers—or clean the containers with disinfectant wipes yourself.

defenses. Of course, convincing kids—especially finicky ones—to eat good-for-them foods can be a challenge. These tips can help.

Ply them with produce. Fruits and vegetables are packed with antioxidants that will fuel kids' immune systems through cold and flu season, says Laura Jeffers, RD, a pediatric dietitian at Cleveland Clinic in Ohio. But what if the only green that your child will eat is lime Jell-O?

✚ Offer fun-to-eat finger foods like baby carrots, berries, and orange and tangerine slices. You can increase the fun factor by adding something for dunking, like low-fat salad dressing for the veggies or fruit dip for the berries.

✚ Top steamed broccoli with melted cheese (fat-free or 1 or 2 % milk) for a surefire kid-pleaser.

✚ Offer vegetable juice as a beverage—or, if that isn't appealing, try one of the new veggie-fruit combo juices, such as V8 V-Fusion.

+ Make a fruit smoothie by combining frozen fruit such as strawberries, blueberries, and sliced bananas with yogurt (plain or flavored) and orange juice. Blend until smooth.

+ If your child flat-out refuses to eat veggies, go the surreptitious route by pureeing them and mixing them into more palatable fare. Jeffers suggests coordinating colors to make the disguise complete. For example, try adding pureed roasted cauliflower with mac 'n' cheese, or pureed carrots to spaghetti sauce. Those fussy taste buds won't know the difference.

Stock the fridge with yogurt. Yogurt contains beneficial bacteria, which can help protect against gastrointestinal bugs. Look for a brand that contains live, active cultures—it should say so on the label—and contains no more than 120 calories in a 4- to 6-ounce serving.

Trade sugary drinks for green tea. Like fruits and veggies, green tea is a good source of immune-friendly antioxidants. You can brew your own at home or look for iced green tea at the supermarket. Just make sure that it's "diet" or "sugar-free"; some brands contain as much sugar—and as many calories—as an equal amount of soda.

Fill in gaps with a multivitamin. If your child has a limited diet and eats only certain foods, a kid's multivitamin can help make up for any nutritional shortfalls, Jeffers says.

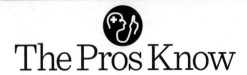

The Pros Know

Sarah Kemeter
Elementary school art teacher in Pike Creek, Delaware

The job of teacher ranks highest on the list of germiest professions. Here's what elementary art teacher Ms. Kemeter does to keep herself well:

Staying away from germs during cold and flu season is really tough. My students, especially the younger ones, constantly want to hug me and get close. It's hard not to hug back!

To stay healthy, I take a multivitamin, and I suck on one or two vitamin C drops during school days. I also exercise regularly, usually six to seven times a week. And I eat well—lots of fruits and vegetables and a few cups of green tea a day.

While at school, I wash my hands a lot—probably at least five times a day, not counting after using the restroom. I also keep hand sanitizer on my desk and use it throughout the day, particularly after I've been in contact with a child who looks like he or she may be sick.

The kids do their part, too. I have them clean their tables every few days with Clorox disinfectant wipes, and I encourage them to use the hand sanitizer.

Index

Underscored page references indicate sidebars.